This book sets out a weight-loss programme.

The programme should not be undertaken by
anyone with an underlying health issue without the
consultation/advice of their regular medical adviser
or a medical professional familiar with their medical
history. In the event of adverse or unusual symptoms
medical advice should be obtained immediately from
a medical doctor or other healthcare provider.

This book is not a substitute for individualized
or personal medical advice and the author and
publisher are not liable for any adverse consequences
of following this weight-loss/diet programme.

The Dukan Diet

Pierre Dukan

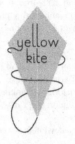

First published in France in 2000 by Flammarion

First published in Great Britain in 2010 by Hodder & Stoughton
An Hachette UK company

Reissued in 2018 by Yellow Kite

This paperback edition published in 2021

4

A CIP catalogue record for this title is available from the British Library

Paperback ISBN 978 1 473 69807 9
eBook ISBN 978 1 473 69809 3

Typeset in Celeste by Hewer Text UK Ltd, Edinburgh
Printed and bound in Great Britain by Clays Ltd, Elcograf S.p.A.

Hodder & Stoughton policy is to use papers that are natural, renewable
and recyclable products and made from wood grown in sustainable
forests. The logging and manufacturing processes are expected to
conform to the environmental regulations of the country of origin.

Yellow Kite
Hodder & Stoughton Ltd
Carmelite House
50 Victoria Embankment
London EC4Y 0DZ

www.yellowkitebooks.co.uk

For Sacha and Maya,
for Maya and Sacha,
my two children,
for the second life they have offered me,
in return for the gift of life I have given to them.

To Christine, my wife,
without whom this endeavour
could never have even been imagined.

To Sylvia and Maurice
who still speak through me.

Contents

Preface

A Decisive Encounter – Or the Man Who Only Liked Meat

My first contact with obesity goes back to the time when, as a very young doctor, I was practising general medicine in the Montparnasse area in Paris, while also specializing in neurology for paraplegic children in Garches, just outside the capital.

At that time, one of my patients was an obese, jovial and tremendously cultivated publisher. I treated him regularly for a very trying case of asthma. One day he came to see me and, once he was seated comfortably in an armchair that creaked under his weight, he said: 'Doctor, I have always been satisfied with your treatment. I trust you, and I've come to see you today because I want you to make me lose weight.'

In those days, all I knew about nutrition and obesity was what my teachers had passed on at medical school, which amounted to simply suggesting low-calorie diets and miniature-sized meals that in every respect looked normal but whose portions were so tiny that any obese person would smile and run a mile. For big eaters, used to living life to the full, the very idea of having to ration their happiness is preposterous.

I declined, stuttering under the pretext that I knew nothing of the subtleties of this science.

'What science are you talking about? I have seen every specialist in Paris, everyone who'd put me on a starvation diet. Since my teens I've lost over seven hundred pounds and I've put it all back on again. I have to admit that I have never been deeply motivated and without realizing it my wife has done me no great service by loving me despite all my extra pounds. I can't find any clothes that fit and, if I'm honest, I'm beginning to fear for my life.'

He then finished off with this last sentence which, alone, changed the course of my professional life: 'Put me on whatever diet you want, deprive me of whatever food you want, anything, but not meat, I like meat too much.'

And I can still remember how I replied without the slightest hesitation:

'Fine, since you like meat so much, come back tomorrow on an empty stomach and weigh yourself on my scales. For the next five days eat nothing but meat. However, avoid fatty meats like pork, lamb, and the fattier cuts of beef such as ribs or rib eye. Grill your meat and drink as much water as you can. Then come back in five days' time on an empty stomach and weigh yourself again.'

'OK, you have a deal.'

Five days later, he was back. He had lost almost 12 pounds. I couldn't believe my eyes and neither could he. I felt somewhat concerned, but he looked great, more jovial than ever, saying he had rediscovered his wellbeing and had stopped snoring. He brushed aside my hesitations.

'I'll keep it up. I feel on top of the world; it works and it is a real treat.'

And so he left for another five days of eating meat, promising me he would have blood and urine tests done.

When he came back, he had lost another five pounds and, jubilant, he showed me his test results. The levels were all perfectly normal: no sugar, no cholesterol and no uric acid.

In the meantime I had gone to the medical school library where I spent time learning more about the nutritional characteristics of meat, extending my research into the great family of proteins, whose most prestigious member is meat.

So, when he returned five days later, still in tip-top shape and having shed another four pounds, I told him to add fish and seafood, which he accepted with good grace because he had explored all that meat had to offer.

When at the end of the first 20 days the scales registered a loss of 22 pounds, he did another blood test that turned out to be just as reassuring as the first one. Playing my ace, I had him add the remaining categories of protein that I still had left, throwing in together dairy products, poultry and eggs. However, to allay my concerns, I asked him to increase his water intake to three litres – about five pints – a day.

He then finally gave in and agreed to add vegetables, as I was beginning to worry that they had been absent from his diet for so long.

When he came back five days later he had not lost an

ounce. He used this as an argument to request going back to his favourite diet with all the categories of proteins he had developed a taste for, especially when he could eat as much of them as he liked. I let him have his way but on condition that he alternated this diet with five-day periods that would include vegetables, arguing that otherwise he risked vitamin deficiency, which he did not buy at all. However, he agreed to add vegetables because he was suffering from constipation, due to the lack of fibre in his diet.

This is how my alternative protein diet was born, as well as my interest in obesity and all categories of excessive weight gain. It changed the course of my studies and my professional life. Having opened my own practice, I patiently worked with this diet, constantly improving it and moulding it to create an eating plan that seems to me today to be both the most appropriate for the particular psychological make-up of overweight people and also the most efficient for weight loss based on real food.

However, over the years, I have come to the bitter realization that weight-loss diets do not stand the test of time, even when effective and followed properly. Lacking real stabilization, their results fade away, at best as a slow and imperceptible drifting off course, at worst the weight piles back on again usually due to stress, setbacks or other problems.

It was seeing how the vast majority of dieters inevitably lose this war against weight that led me to design a diet that consolidates the target weight, a bastion of defence against early setbacks and against the demoralization of regaining lost pounds that leads to self-loathing, to giving it all up and to putting loads of weight back on. The job of this protective stage is to reintroduce, in successive layers, the basic elements of proper eating and I designed it to control a body that, stripped of its reserves, would be bent on revenge. And, to allow enough time for this rebellious phase and to make the transition acceptable, I fixed a precise time limit for this diet, easy to calculate and in proportion to the weight lost: five days for every pound lost.

But, here again, once the consolidation test was over, I saw old habits gradually creep back with the help of the pressures of metabolism: above all, the inevitable resurgence of our need to compensate for life's miseries with those thick, creamy, sweet comfort foods that craftily overwhelm our defences.

To put an end to this once and for all, I had to resort to a measure that is hard to even suggest to people, a rule that I dare call 'permanent', the kind of shackle that all overweight people – the obese of whatever size, or the just plain chubby – detest and reject *a priori* because it is there for good. It goes against the grain, and their need to be impulsive and their absolute horror of being supervised. This rule, to be followed for the rest of one's life but which guarantees real stabilization, is unacceptable unless it applies to only a single day a week, a day that is predetermined, whose structure cannot be changed or negotiated but which bears amazing results.

It was only then that I reached the Promised Land: genuine, long-lasting, unequivocal success built on a quartet of successive diets, each decreasing in intensity, which time and experience had led me to interweave with each other to create a supportive and clearly signposted path that allows no escape. A short, strict Attack diet but with lightning results, followed by a Cruise diet alternating between forward thrusts and breaks, sustained by a Consolidation stage, whose duration is proportionate to the weight lost. Finally, so that the weight you have achieved with such effort remains stable forever, there is a locking measure that is as specific as it is effective: a single day once a week devoted to dietary redemption, to keep the rest of the week in balance, provided it stays by your side, like a loyal guard dog, for the rest of your life.

Finally I achieved my first real lasting results. Now I no longer had only a fish to offer, but a whole course on how to fish, a comprehensive programme that allowed overweight people to be autonomous, lose weight quickly and keep it off for good, and to do this all by themselves.

I have spent over 40 years creating this beautiful tool by hand for a limited number of people. Today with my pen I want a wider public to be able to access my programme and its interconnected diets.

This programme is intended for those of you who have tried everything, who have lost weight often – too often – and who are looking for a way not just to lose weight, but more importantly to maintain those hard-earned results and live comfortably with the body you want and deserve. This is what I am offering you, in exchange for the effort that for a limited period of time you agree to make and keep up without fail.

So I dedicate this book and this method to all my patients who were won over by my direct, verbal advice, to my patients and clients who have made my life as a doctor so fulfilling, my flesh and blood people, young and old, men and women, and in particular the very first of them, the overweight publisher.

THE BIRTH OF A FOUR-STEP DIET

The Dukan Diet

Over 40 years have passed since the decisive encounter with the obese gentleman who changed the course of my life. Since then, I have devoted my work to nutrition and to helping the fat and the not-so-fat lose pounds and stabilize their weight.

Like all my French medical colleagues, I was trained with Cartesian measure and balance as the rule, where calories were counted and low-calorie diets taught, every type of food was allowed but in moderate quantities.

As soon as I arrived on the scene, this neat theory – based on the crazy hope that it was possible to reprogramme overweight people and their eating excesses and turn them into methodical calorie-counters – exploded into smithereens. Nowadays, what I know and practise I have learned and developed through direct daily contact with flesh and blood human beings, with men, but more often women, who have constant cravings to eat.

So I very quickly realized that it was not by accident that a fat individual was overweight; that their gourmet appetite, their gluttony and apparent lack of restraint was a camouflage concealing a need to find comfort in food and that this need is all the more overwhelming as it is connected to our survival mechanisms, which are as archaic as they are instinctive.

It soon became obvious to me that you could not make an overweight person lose weight and stay slim simply by giving them sound advice, even if that advice is based on common sense or scientific research, as the person has no other choice but to obey or try to wriggle out of it.

Support is what an overweight person determined to lose weight really wants and what they need from a counsellor or a method; support so that they are not left alone to face the ordeal of dieting, which deliberately goes against their own instinct for survival.

So what the overweight individual is looking for is an outside will, a decision-maker, who walks on ahead of them offering guidance, providing them with instructions, more instructions and ever more instructions, because what the overweight individual most hates and simply cannot do is decide for themselves when and how they are going to deprive themselves of food.

As for managing their weight, an overweight person will admit without shame – and why should there be any? – that they are weak and even immature. I have known all kinds of overweight people, from every social background, ordinary people to the great and good, executives, bankers, even politicians, intelligent people, brilliant and eminent people, but who have all sat there in front of me and described themselves as being astonishingly weak when it comes to food, using it like a greedy child and unable to stop themselves.

Obviously, most of them, from early childhood onwards, have found in food an easy 'escape valve', through which they can release excess tension, stress and life's all too frequent disappointments. So any logical, reasonable and rational instructions cannot stand up to, or not for long, the pressures of the body's archaic system of defence.

During my years of practice, I have seen all the diets come and go that have hit the headlines and marked their era and this has only reinforced my convictions. Since the early 1950s I have counted more than 200 such diets, some of them promoted and popularized by books that became worldwide successes, selling millions of copies, diets such as the Atkins, the Scarsdale, the Montignac and the Weight Watchers. These examples of typical diet books brought home to me just how much an overweight individual welcomes with open arms such regimes with their built-in instructions.

Analyzing these diets and the reasons behind their incredible success, as well as my own practice and my daily contact with overweight people, observing the strength of their resolve at certain times in their lives and then seeing how easily they lose heart when the results do not match their efforts, all this has convinced me that:

An overweight person who wants to lose weight needs a fast-acting diet that brings immediate results, fast enough to strengthen and maintain their motivation, and they also need precise goals to achieve, set by an outside instructor, with a series of various levels and crossing points to aim for so that they can see their efforts and compare them with the results expected.

Most of the spectacular diets that rocketed to success in recent years did in fact have that fast-off-the-mark effect and delivered the promised results. Unfortunately, their instructions, guidance and the levels or stages faded away once the book was read, leaving the overweight individual once again all alone on a slippery slope to confront their temptations. As the same causes lead to the same effects, the cycle would start all over again. Once the goal was reached, all these diets, even the most original and inventive, so far as the Attack phase goes, turned out to be strangely mediocre. They abandoned their followers with the same old common-sense advice about moderation and balance that an ex-overweight person will never manage to follow.

None of these famous diets has managed to find a way of protecting and guiding the individual during the period that follows their weight loss, of giving advice and precise, simple and effective landmarks, just like those that had made their Attack phase so successful.

The overweight person, who has lost weight and feels victorious, knows instinctively that on their own and without any support they will not be able to preserve this victory. They also know that left to their own devices the pounds will go back on, slowly at first, then more quickly, as they do nothing by halves.

The overweight person who has just lost weight using a method that told them what to do needs a reminder of that symbolic presence or of that hand that held theirs and guided them as they lost weight. They need instructions that are simple enough but specific, effective and not too frustrating so that they can be followed for the rest of their life.

Dissatisfied with the majority of the main diets in vogue, which are only concerned with a dazzling but short-lived victory, and aware of how ineffective low-calorie diets are and common-sense advice that despite all the evidence hopes to reform overeaters into careful eaters, I developed my own weight-loss diet: the alternating protein diet. This book explains my diet, which years of medical practice allow me to consider as being both the most effective and easy-to-follow diet available today. I realize that put this way I may appear immodest. But I will take that risk because it is my most heartfelt conviction and not saying so, in the face of the growing scourge of weight-control problems, would amount to a failure to assist people in danger.

This diet, with its first two actual slimming phases, is made up of a pair of diets that work like a two-speed engine, in which a pure protein Attack phase first conquers the field and is then immediately followed by a period when these same proteins are combined with vegetables – a time when the body can recuperate and adjust to its weight loss.

As time went by and noticing how easily my patients'

resolve slackened as soon as their goal was reached and how without any instructions and precise framework they would backslide, this diet gradually turned into a comprehensive weight-loss programme.

My programme takes into account the overweight person's particular psychology and includes everything that is essential for the success of any weight loss which we have just described and which I can sum up as follows:

- The Dukan Diet offers overweight people trying to lose weight a system with specific instructions that get them on track, with stages and objectives, leaving no room for ambiguity or deviation.
- Leaving aside fasting and protein powder diets, of all the diets based on real food that I have had the opportunity of working with, the Dukan Diet is today the one that seems to me to produce the best results. The initial weight loss is substantial and sufficiently rapid to launch the diet and instil lasting motivation.
- The Dukan Diet is a low-frustration diet; weighing food portions and calorie-counting are banned and it allows you total freedom to eat a certain number of popular foods.
- The Dukan Diet is not just a simple diet; it is a comprehensive slimming programme, an integrated whole that you either take or leave. It can be broken down into four successive phases:

The Attack Phase

An initial Attack phase led by the 'pure protein diet', which creates a stunning kick-start, almost as quick as fasting or powdered protein diets but without their drawbacks.

The Cruise Phase

A Cruise phase led by an 'alternating protein diet', when pure protein days alternate with pure proteins + vegetable days, which allows you to reach your chosen weight non-stop in one go.

The Consolidation Phase

When the weight you have achieved is consolidated: a phase designed to prevent the rebound effect that occurs after any rapid weight loss. This is a period of high vulnerability when the body has a tendency to very easily regain those lost pounds. It has a very precise timescale: five days for every pound lost.

The Stabilization Phase

Finally, and most importantly, permanent stabilization based on three simple safety measures that are easy to follow but indispensable if the weight loss is to be maintained: the Dukan Diet has to be followed one set day per week – e.g. every Thursday – for the rest of your life; do not use lifts or escalators; and take three tablespoons of oat bran a day. Three rules that are indeed strict and non-negotiable, but sufficiently specific and effective that you can stick to them over such a long period of time.

The Theory Behind the Dukan Diet

Before looking at the diet in detail and explaining exactly how it works and why it is so effective, I believe it necessary to outline the whole programme with its four-phase structure to make clear to the reader from the outset precisely for whom the diet is intended along with any possible contra-indications.

The Dukan Diet is not only the most reliable and best performing of all current weight-loss diets, it is a more ambitious, comprehensive programme, a four-stage system of instructions with decreasing strictness, which from day one takes complete charge of the overweight person and never, ever, lets them down.

One of the major merits of the Dukan Diet is its educational value. It allows obese people to learn in real life and with their own body the relative importance of each food group based on the order in which they are integrated into their diet. It starts with vital foods, then introduces, in succession, indispensable foods, essential foods and important foods, finishing off with superfluous foods.

The stated objective of the Dukan Diet is to provide a system of perfectly interwoven instructions that are sufficiently clear and direct to set the dieter on the right track, avoiding the need for that never-ending effort of willpower, which slowly undermines their determination.

These instructions join together in four successive

diets, the first two making up the actual weight-loss phase, while the next two ensure that the weight loss achieved is consolidated then permanently stabilized.

The Attack Phase: the Pure Protein Diet

This is the conquest phase when the person starting the diet is extremely motivated. They are looking for a diet which, however arduous it might be, meets their expectations in terms of effectiveness and quick results and allows them to tackle their weight problem head-on.

This initial diet, great for a fast-track approach, is the 'pure protein diet'. Its theoretical goal is to limit food to just one of the three food groups, namely, proteins.

In theory, except for egg whites, no food is 100 per cent protein. This diet therefore selects and groups together foods whose composition is as close as possible to pure protein, such as certain kinds of meat, fish, seafood, poultry, eggs, plant proteins and non-fat dairy products.

Compared to all the low-calorie diets, this diet is a real war-machine, a bulldozer which, if followed without fail, crushes all resistance. It is by far the quickest and best performing of the safe diets based on real food. It is effective in the most difficult cases, in particular for premenopausal women suffering from water retention and swelling or confirmed menopausal women starting the critical period of hormone treatment. It is just as effective with patients deemed to be 'resistant', because they have tried and given up too many diets or aggressive courses of treatment in the past.

The Cruise Phase: the Alternating Protein Diet

As its name indicates, this diet works by alternating two diets, one after the other. The two diets interconnect: the pure protein diet is followed by the same diet to which any green or cooked vegetable is added. Each alternate cycle works like the injection-combustion of a two-speed engine burning up its calorie quota.

Alternating diets

The first and second diets both allow you total freedom with regard to quantities. You can eat the authorized 'as much as you like' foods at any time of day and in the combination and quantity that best suits you. This gives you both complete freedom and an effective way of neutralizing your hunger by eating. Satisfaction through quantity makes up for any lack of quality.

Details are given later of the precise timing for the alternating pattern of these two diets depending on how much weight you want to lose, how many diets you have already attempted, your age and level of motivation.

This Attack phase, which often begins with an impressive weight loss, must be followed without a break until your target weight is reached. Although influenced in part by previous bad experiences, the alternating protein diet is still one of the diets least affected by resistance induced by previous attempts at weight loss.

Consolidating the Weight Obtained: Five Days for Every Pound Lost

After the conquest phase comes the soothing phase of the Dukan Diet. Its essential purpose is to get you eating necessary foods again, while avoiding the traditional rebound effect that occurs after losing a lot of weight. Throughout the Attack phase and in an increasingly obvious manner as the diet continues, the body tries to put up resistance. It reacts to its reserves being plundered by gradually reducing its energy output and, above all, by assimilating and getting as much energy as possible from any food that is eaten.

The triumphant fat person is therefore sitting on a volcano: their body is just waiting for the right moment to win back its lost reserves. A large meal that before the diet would have had little effect will now, towards the end of the diet, have far-reaching consequences.

This is why the diet opens up to include foods that are richer and more gratifying, but their variety and quantity will be limited, so that the body's metabolism can calm down, without running any risk, after it has worked so hard to lose weight.

So, two slices of bread and one portion of fruit and cheese are introduced per day, along with two servings of carbohydrates and, above all, two 'celebration' meals a week.

The purpose of this first Stabilization stage is, therefore, to avoid the explosive rebound that is the most immediate and one of the most frequent reasons for failure in weight-loss diets. It is now necessary to introduce foods as significant as bread, fruit, cheese and some starches as well as access to certain superfluous but extremely pleasurable dishes or foods. They must, however, be introduced in a certain order, with a set of instructions that are sufficiently precise and supportive to avoid the continual risk of slipping backwards. The role of this first bastion is to protect the weight loss. How long this phase lasts depends on how much has been lost; a very simple calculation based on five days for every pound lost.

Ultimate Long-term Stabilization

Having lost weight and avoided any rebound by using the reassuring system of instructions and accepting certain constraints, the triumphant and often euphoric fat person knows instinctively that their victory is fragile and that, without support, sooner or later – and more often sooner rather than later – they will be at the mercy of their old demons. One thing they are even more certain of is that they will never acquire the moderation and measure when it comes to food that most nutritionists rightly recommend as the way guaranteed to maintain this weight loss. In this fourth phase, the Dukan Diet offers the dieter the original Attack phase, the pure protein diet, both its most effective and strictest weapon, once a week, every Thursday, for the rest of their life.

As paradoxical as this might seem, once the fat person has reached their desired weight, they are quite capable of making this effort one day a week because it is a very precise rule and lasts a very limited amount of time. And, above all, this specific and non-negotiable rule bears immediate fruit but allows the dieter to eat normally for the other six days of the week without putting any weight back on.

The Dukan Diet summarized

1. *The Attack diet: Pure Proteins*
Average length: five days

2. *The Cruise diet: 100 unlimited foods in alternation*
Average length: three days for each pound you want to lose

3. *The Consolidation diet*
Average length: five days per pound lost

4. *The Stabilization diet*
One pure protein day every Thursday for life
No more lifts and escalators
3 tablespoons of oatbran a day

SOME USEFUL INFORMATION ABOUT NUTRITION

The CLP Trio: Carbohydrates – Lipids – Proteins

A ll food, whether for humans or animals, provides an impressive number of edible foodstuffs, but these are all made up of only three nutrients: carbohydrates, lipids and proteins. Every food gets its taste, texture and nutritional interest from the particular way that these three elements combine.

Calories Are Unequal in Quality

Once upon a time, nutritional experts were only interested in the calorific value of foods and meals and they based their weight-loss diets entirely on calorie-counting, which explains why for so long they failed without any apparent explanation.

Today, most of them have abandoned this approach based exclusively on quantity and instead are more interested in where the calories come from, the type of food providing them, the mix of nutrients that makes up the mass of chewed food and even the time of day when the calories are taken in.

It can be proved today that the body does not treat 100 calories provided by white sugar in the same way as it does 100 calories from oil or fish, and that the ultimate benefit of these calories after they are assimilated varies widely, depending on their origin.

The same holds true for the time of day they are eaten. Although disputed in the past, it is now commonly agreed that the body burns up morning calories better than midday calories and even better than evening calories. Leaving aside the fact that it is specifically adapted to the overweight person's specific profile, the effectiveness of the Dukan Diet's four-diet plan can be explained by the very careful selection of nutrients that make up the foods we recommend, in particular the huge importance given to proteins during the Attack phase as well as during long-term stabilization.

It is very important, therefore, especially for anyone who does not have much knowledge of nutrition, to compare these three food groups so that the original way in which my programme works can be better understood.

Carbohydrates

This very widespread and much enjoyed food category has always supplied man, whatever the place, era or culture, with over 50 per cent of his energy ration.

For thousands of years, apart from fruit and honey, the only carbohydrates consumed by man were what we nowadays call 'slow sugars': cereal grains, starches, legumes, etc. What sets them apart is that they are absorbed gradually and sugar levels are only moderately raised, thus preventing insulin surges in reaction and the harmful repercussions on health and specifically on weight gain that we nowadays recognize.

Since we discovered how to extract white sugar from sugar cane and then from sugar beet, human food has undergone profound changes, with our ever-increasing intake of sweet foods and quick-penetration carbohydrates. Providing excellent fuel, carbohydrates are highly suitable for athletes, manual workers and teenagers. But for the vast majority of sedentary people who make up most of today's societies they are far from useful.

- White sugar and all its derivatives, such as confectionery and sweets, are pure carbohydrates, rich and absorbed in no time at all.
- Starchy foods, even if they do not taste sweet, are just as rich in carbohydrates. They include flour products (bread, in particular white bread, crackers, biscuits, cereals, etc.), pasta, potatoes, peas, legumes, lentils and beans.
- The fruit containing the most carbohydrates are bananas, cherries and grapes.
- Wine and all alcohol.
- Pastries – they are a delicious combination of flour and sugar, and, even worse, of fat.

Carbohydrates contain only four calories per gram, but usually their intake is large so the calories soon mount up. They are also totally assimilated, which increases their energy yield. Furthermore, we digest starch and flour products slowly, producing fermentation and gas, which causes swelling as unpleasant as it is unattractive.

Whether starch, flour products or sweet-tasting, most carbohydrates are very popular. Our affinity for sweet tastes is in part innate, but most psychologists agree that lengthy conditioning starting in childhood makes sweet flavours gratifying as they are associated with rewards.

Finally, carbohydrates are almost always the cheapest foods available, which is why they are served at everyone's table from the richest to the poorest. In conclusion, carbohydrates are foods that are both energy-rich and found everywhere and have such a pleasant taste that they are often used as comfort foods. And as for sweet foods, some people snack on them compulsively.

As far as the body's metabolism is concerned, carbohydrates help the secretion of insulin which in turn encourages fat to be produced and stored. For all these reasons, for a long time anyone predisposed to being overweight traditionally had to be wary of carbohydrates. More recently, they were told instead to be wary of the fat content in foods, which – and rightly so – became the overweight person's most deadly enemy. However, this is not a reason to lower one's guard, especially during the Attack phase, which has to be as high-performing and rapid as possible. The Dukan Diet excludes carbohydrates completely during the Attack phase. In the Cruise phase and until the desired weight has been reached, it only allows vegetables with extremely low sugar levels. Carbohydrates make a comeback during the Consolidation phase but it is only during the final Stabilization phase, six days out of seven, that total restriction is lifted.

Lipids

Lipids (fats) are the absolute enemy of anyone trying to be slim as they represent, for every living species, the most concentrated form in which surplus energy is stored. Eating fats means you are eating an animal's fat reserves, which, in theory as in practice, stands every chance of increasing your weight.

Since the Atkins diet appeared, opening the way for lipids by demonizing carbohydrates, many diets have adopted this sensationalized point of view, which served its promoter so well. It was quite clearly a major mistake, and for two reasons: cholesterol and triglyceride levels rise dangerously, some people paying for this with their lives; and mistrust of fats is gone and once gone it makes any form of stabilization impossible.

There are two major sources of lipids: animal fat and vegetable fat. Animal fat, found in a virtually pure state in lard, is very much present in pork products such as pâtés, salamis, sausages, hot-dogs, meat spreads, etc. But a number of other animals also supply it. Lamb and mutton and certain poultry, such as goose and duck, have a plentiful supply. Beef is not as fatty, especially those cuts that can be grilled. Only ribs and the rib eye are really rich in fat. Butter, which comes from the creamy top of milk, is practically a pure lipid. Fresh cream, which contains more water, is nonetheless fatty and its lipid content is around 80 per cent.

Among fish, there are five main sources of fat, easily recognizable by their rich taste and blue skin: sardines, tuna, salmon, mackerel and herring. But remember that as fatty as these five fish are, they are no fattier than ordinary steak and, above all, the fat of cold-water fish is rich in omega-3 fatty acids, a known safeguard against cardiovascular disease.

Vegetable lipids are for the most part represented by the long list of oils and the family of oleaginous fruits. Oil is even fattier than butter. And if some oils like olive, rapeseed or sunflower have nutritional qualities that have been proven to protect the heart and arteries, they all have the same calorific value and should be banned from any weight-loss diet, avoided during the Consolidation phase and eaten sparingly during the final Stabilization phase. As for oleaginous foods – peanuts, walnuts, hazelnuts, pistachios, etc. – these are automatic snack foods often eaten with an aperitif, and the combination with alcohol greatly increases the calorie intake of the meal to follow.

For those who want to be slim or, in particular, for those who are trying to lose weight, lipids represent every danger possible.

- They contain, by far, the most calories: nine calories per gram (more than double carbohydrates, which provide only four calories per gram).

- Lipids are very rich foods and so are rarely eaten alone. Oil, butter and fresh cream are often associated with bread, starch, pasta or vinaigrette: the combination increases the overall calorie count considerably.
- Fats are not assimilated as quickly as fast sugars, but far more quickly than proteins, and so their comparative energy contribution increases accordingly.
- Fatty foods only reduce our appetite moderately and snacking on them, rather than proteins, does not reduce our desire for a large meal afterwards, or delay the time before you next feel hungry.
- Finally, animal lipids – butter, sausages, dried meats and fat cheeses – with high amounts of fatty acids, pose a potential threat to the heart. For this reason, they cannot be consumed without restriction, as has been the case with the Atkins diet and other regimes inspired by it.

Proteins

Proteins are the third universal food group. They form a large group of nitrogenous substances and have the longest molecules that exist in living beings. The foods richest in proteins come from the animal kingdom. Their most prestigious source is meat.

Among animal meat, beef is especially high in protein. The leaner cuts are extremely low in fat, but just as rich in protein. Mutton and lamb are visibly more marbled and this infiltration of fat, which tones down their colour, reduces their protein content. Finally, pork, which is even fattier, is not rich enough in protein to belong to the elite group of essentially protein foods.

Kidneys, liver, tongue, sweetbreads, chicken hearts and tripe are very rich in protein, and low in fat and carbohydrates. However, liver contains a small dose of sugar.

Poultry, with the exception of domestic goose and duck, is a relatively lean meat very rich in protein, especially turkey and chicken breast.

Fish, namely lean white fish like sole, skate, cod, sea bass or hake, are a gold mine of proteins with a very high biological value. Cold-water fish such as salmon, tuna, sardines or mackerel have fattier flesh which slightly reduces their protein content, but they nevertheless remain excellent sources of protein, have a delicate and appealing taste and greatly promote cardiovascular health.

Shellfish and other types of seafood are lean and carbohydrate-free and therefore rich in protein. Some, like scallops, are often not allowed because of their high cholesterol level, but that substance is concentrated in the coral of the animal's head and not its flesh, which means that you can eat prawns, crab and other seafood without restriction, as long as you take the precaution of removing the coral first.

Eggs are an interesting source of protein. The yolk contains lipids and enough cholesterol that should you be predisposed to high cholesterol excessive consumption should be avoided. On the other hand, egg white is the purest and most complete known form of protein, which gives it the status of benchmark protein, as it is used to classify all other proteins.

Proteins are not exclusive to the animal kingdom; we can find a lot of proteins in the plant kingdom too. However, these plant proteins are incomplete and never contain all eight essential amino acids, without which they cannot be digested by the human body. As it happens, cereals are rich in all amino acids except just one: lysine, whereas legumes do have lysine, but they in turn have no methionine, which is found in abundance in cereals. You'll have grasped then that if you want to eat plant proteins you'll have to mix them together in equal quantities. Furthermore, although animal proteins contain a little fat, by choosing carefully you can find some really lean ones. Plant proteins, on the other hand, usually have a fairly high carbohydrate content, so you'll need to restrict your intake and choose those with the least carbohydrate, such as pasta or lentils.

So how can we be vegetarian? It all depends on how this word is defined. If it means just cutting out all red meat, there are many other sources of animal protein such as fish, seafood, eggs and dairy products that can provide an ample intake. If it means not eating anything from an animal that has been raised and slaughtered for us to eat then it becomes more difficult, as this leaves only eggs and dairy products, but this is possible and sufficient for people who are not trying to lose weight. If vegetarian means only eating vegetables, my diet becomes very hard to follow as there is no other choice but to use incomplete plant proteins. These have to be very cleverly teamed up with cereals and leguminous plants to ensure that all amino acids are consumed because without all of them, it is impossible to produce vital proteins.

Man is a carnivorous hunter

It is important to realise that man emerged from his animal condition by becoming carnivorous. His ape-like ancestors, like today's great anthropoid apes, were essentially vegetarians, even if, occasionally, certain apes did hunt other animals for food. Indeed it was by becoming a group hunter and therefore a meat-eater that man was able to acquire purely human faculties. The human body possesses a whole system for digestion and elimination that still allows us today to eat unlimited quantities of meat and fish.

We are designed to eat animals, meat, fish and poultry, as far as both our metabolism and psychology are concerned. Yes, we can get by without them and it is possible to live without hunting and without eating animal meat BUT by doing so we give up a part of what our nature expects and we lessen the emotional effect that our body is programmed to produce when we give it what it expects. What I am saying to you here may seem trivial but it is absolutely crucial, as the purpose of any living creature, whether animal or human, is to live in such a way that what it does fits with why it has been made that way.

Digestion, calorie loss and satisfaction

Of all the food categories, the digestion of proteins is the longest and most laborious. It takes over three hours to break down and assimilate proteins. The reason for this is simple. Their molecules are long chains with well-soldered links and to break down their resistance requires the combination of good chewing, laborious processing in the stomach and in particular the simultaneous attack of various gastric, pancreatic and biliary juices.

This long process of calorie extraction greatly taxes the system and it has been calculated that to obtain 100 calories from a protein food, 30 have to be used up. This particular feature can be summed up by saying that the specific dynamic action of proteins is 30 per cent, while it is only 12 per cent for lipids and just 7 per cent for carbohydrates.

What we should remember from this is that when someone wanting to lose weight consumes meat, fish or non-fat yoghurt, the person has to work hard simply to digest and assimilate the food, and the calories they use doing this reduces the energy intake from the meal. This really works in the favour of anyone wanting to lose weight. We will explore this at greater length when we explain how the pure protein diet works. What is more, this slow rate of digestion and assimilation delays gastric drainage and increases our sense of 'feeling full' and of satisfaction.

The only vital and indispensable nutrient at every meal

Of the three universal food groups, only proteins are

indispensable for our existence. Of these three groups, carbohydrates are the least necessary because our bodies can produce glucose, i.e. sugar, from meat or fat. This is what happens when we are deprived of food or are dieting: we draw upon our fat reserves, transforming them into the glucose that is vital for our muscles and brain. The same goes for lipids: with their excessive intake of sugars and meat an obese person is expert in both making and storing them.

On the other hand, man does not have the metabolic means to synthesize proteins. The simple fact of being alive, of ensuring that our muscular system is maintained, red blood cells renewed, that wounds heal, hair grows and even that memory functions, all these vital operations require proteins, a minimum of one gram per day for every two pounds of body weight.

Whenever there is a shortage, the body is forced to draw upon its reserves, mainly its muscles, but it also uses its skin or even its bones. This is what happens if unreasonable diets are followed, such as water-based liquid fasting with nothing else, or the Beverly Hills diet based entirely on exotic fruits and made famous by Hollywood stars, who must have lost much of their powers of seduction if they really did follow it.

A method called detox, or detox diet, which came from the States, has led people to believe that our bodies can be detoxified by eating just fruit and vegetables for a few days. When you realize it has been scientifically proven that after eight hours without good-quality proteins the body has to draw upon its own muscle reserves to ensure its vital functions, you can understand just how inappropriate such ideas are. They are nothing more than a marketing ploy and a distraction from the real issues.

Anyone wanting to lose weight should therefore realize that however restrictive the diet, it should never supply the body with less than one gram of protein per day for every two pounds of body weight and, most importantly, protein intake should be evenly distributed over the day's three meals. A meagre breakfast, lunch consisting of a pastry and a bar of chocolate, then pizza for dinner with fruit for dessert are all meals that lack protein and will make your skin dull and impair your body's general strength.

The low-calorie value of proteins

A gram of protein provides only four calories, the same as sugar, but half of what fat provides. Still, the great difference lies in the fact that the concentration of proteins in protein-rich foods is never as high as that of carbohydrates in table sugar, or of lipids in oil or butter.

Only 50 per cent of all meat, fish and other food proteins are assimilated, the rest is waste or useless tissue. Therefore, 115g (4oz) of turkey or steak provides only 200 calories and when you take into account that your body has to contribute 30 per cent of this calorific value, that is, 60 calories, just to assimilate it, only 140 calories are left from this tasty and filling food – the equivalent of a tablespoon of the dressing that you deem so harmless as you add it to your salad.

These simple facts show you the vital importance of using a diet that dares, for a limited period, to offer only proteins.

Two drawbacks regarding proteins:

- They are expensive: the cost of protein is relatively high – meat, fish and seafood can easily make a dent in a modest budget. Eggs, poultry and offal are more affordable, but still remain expensive. Fortunately, for some time now, with the availability of non-fat dairy products it has been possible to get excellent quality protein at a price that allows us to offset the high cost of protein meals.
- Food high in waste: unlike most other foods, protein foods are not completely broken down. During their digestion, a certain number of waste products, such as uric acid, remain in the system and have to be eliminated. In theory, eating more of these foods would increase the amount of waste products and cause discomfort to anyone who is predisposed or sensitive to such problems. In fact, the human organs, and particularly the kidneys, have a certain number of mechanisms for elimination and are perfectly suited to this task. But to work efficiently, it is absolutely necessary that the kidneys have an increased quantity of water. The kidneys will filter and remove uric acid from our blood, provided that we increase our normal consumption of water.

I had the opportunity to review 60 cases of patients suffering from either gout or uric acid stones. They followed a protein-rich diet and also agreed to drink three litres of water a day. Those who were already following treatment continued with it; the others, who had none, did not add any medication. During the diet there was not a single case of uric acid levels rising; in fact a third of the patients saw their levels go down.

It is therefore essential when following a protein-rich diet to keep drinking water, especially during the protein-only phase. This is an opportune moment to deal with the accusations levelled against proteins by those eternal grumpy old rumour mongers who spread the idea that protein-rich foods can strain and even damage the kidneys. These same spoilsports have extended their attack by stating that even water can be toxic for the kidneys if you drink one and a half litres per day. In more than 40 years of working with my diet and its unrestricted protein intake and insisting that my patients must drink at least a litre and a half per day, I have never had anyone question this. I have even worked with 30 patients who, despite having only one kidney, lost weight without ever noting any change in their renal markers. Apart from the usual prophets of doom, there are also jealous and mischievous people, and in particular some people who could do with losing weight themselves but lack the will to do so, who try to stop others from having a go. To such people I say come and join us, and let's drink together!

Conclusion

Let's highlight some of the fundamental principles of a good weight-loss diet:

- Without doubt, lipids or fat both from animals and plants are the greatest enemy for anyone about to embark on a weight-loss diet. Even before you start considering the lipid content in meat or fish, just adding up the calories from the lipids in cooking oil, sauces, marinades, dips, butter, cream, as well as the fat found in cheese and sausages, is enough for lipids to be awarded the prize for the highest source of calories. Therefore an effective, consistent diet has to start by reducing or eliminating lipid-rich foods. You cannot lose your own fat by eating fat from other sources!

- You must also realize that animal fats alone contain cholesterol and triglycerides. They therefore need to be reduced if there is any likelihood of cardiovascular risk or hypercholesterolaemia.

- For anyone wanting to lose weight the simple carbohydrate is their other enemy. Not the slow sugars found in wholegrains or legumes, but fast sugar and table sugar, which are often assimilated instantaneously and whose very presence encourages the rest of the food to be absorbed. A great substance to snack on, the sweet taste can make you forget just how high the calorie concentration is.

- Proteins have a moderate caloric value: four calories per gram.
- Those foods richest in proteins like meat or fish are interwoven with conjunctive tissue, very resistant to digestion, which means they are not completely assimilated. For an overweight person, who by definition is a great calorie assimilator getting the most out of anything they eat, this is manna from heaven as it means they cannot extract all the calories.
- The dynamic action specific to proteins is equal to the calories used to break them down during digestion. Subtract the energy used for digestion from the energy they contribute and an additional 30 per cent is saved, far more than all other foods.
- Never go on a diet with fewer than 50–85g (2–3oz) of pure protein as it will rob you of muscle tissue and make your skin dull.
- Do not worry about uric acid, protein's natural waste product. You will eliminate it entirely by drinking an extra litre and a half of water a day.
- Remember that the slower a food is assimilated, the longer it takes for you to feel hungry again. Sweet foods are absorbed and assimilated the most rapidly, then fatty foods and, only after them, proteins. Those of you who constantly have food on your mind can draw your own conclusions.

PURE PROTEINS

The Driving Force Behind the Dukan Diet

The Dukan Diet programme is made up of four successive interconnected diets designed so that they guide the overweight person to their desired weight and keep them there. These four successive diets, which gradually include more foods, have been specially devised to bring about, in the following order:

- With the first diet, a lightning start and an intense and stimulating weight loss.
- With the second diet, a steady, regular weight loss that takes you straight to your desired weight, your own True Weight.
- With the third diet, consolidation of this newly achieved but still unstable weight, lasting for a fixed period of time – five days for every pound lost.
- With the fourth diet, permanent stabilization, in return for three simple, concrete, guiding, extremely effective but non-negotiable measures to be followed for the rest of your life: protein Thursdays, no more lifts or escalators and three tablespoons of oat bran *a day.*

Each of these diets has a specific effect and a particular mission to accomplish, but all four draw their force and their graduated impact from using pure proteins: pure proteins only during the Attack phase; the proteins are combined with vegetables during the Cruise phase; then they are eaten with other foods during consolidation, and, finally, they are pure again in permanent stabilization but only for one day a week.

The Attack phase gets its jump-start, taking the body by surprise, by using the protein diet in its purest form without compromise, for two to seven days, depending on the individual.

It is this same diet that, by alternating proteins, gives power and rhythm to the Cruise phase, which leads you straight to your desired weight.

It is also this same diet, used occasionally, that is the mainstay of the Consolidation phase, the period of transition between hard-line dieting and a return to normal eating.

And finally it is this diet that, for just one day a week but for the rest of your life, guarantees permanent stabilization. In exchange for this occasional effort, for the other six days of the week you will be able to eat without guilt or any particular restriction.

If the group of 72 protein-rich foods is the driving force behind my programme and its four successive diets, before you put this into practice, and so that you benefit from all it can offer, we need to describe the particular way this diet works and explain its impressive effectiveness.

How does the pure protein diet work? All will be explained in this chapter.

THIS DIET PROVIDES ONLY PROTEINS

Where Do You Find Pure Proteins?

Proteins form the fabric of living matter, both animal and vegetable, so they are found in most known foods. But to develop its unique action and full potential, the protein diet has to be composed of elements as close as possible to pure protein. In practice, other than egg whites, no food is this pure.

Whatever their protein content, in nature vegetables are systematically associated with carbohydrates. This holds true for all cereals and starchy foods, legumes and various starchy vegetables, including whole soya beans, known for having high-quality protein but too much fat and carbohydrates. However, there are products produced from soya and wheat that are processed in such a way that their proteins are isolated and concentrated to form foods such as tofu from soya and seitan from wheat. This is the reason why you'll find these new products included on the list of foods you are allowed to eat with my diet. As for other foods that come from plants, such as certain cereals and legumes, because they contain too many carbohydrates they feature only in the version of my diet that is especially adapted for those vegetarians who eat no animal products except eggs and dairy produce.

The same applies to certain foods of animal origin,

more protein-rich than any vegetables, but which are also too high in fat. This is the case with pork, mutton and lamb, some poultry, such as duck and goose, and some cuts of beef and veal.

There are, however, a certain number of foods of animal origin that, without attaining the level of pure protein, come close to it and because of this they will be the main players in the Dukan Diet.

- Beef, except for ribs, spare ribs and cuts used for braising or stewing
- Lean cuts of veal
- Poultry, except for duck and goose
- All fish, including oily fish whose fat helps protect the heart and arteries so they can be included here
- All other seafood
- Eggs, even though the small amount of fat in the yolk taints the purity of the egg white
- Non-fat dairy products. Though very rich in protein and totally fat-free, they may, nevertheless, contain a small amount of lactose, a natural milk sugar found in milk just as fructose is found in fruit. They can, however, remain in the Dukan Diet's strike force because they have little lactose but lots of taste.

How Do Proteins Work?

The purity of proteins reduces the calories they provide
Every animal species feeds on foods made up of a mixture of the only three known food groups: proteins,

carbohydrates and lipids. But for each species, there is a specific ideal proportion for these three food groups. For humans the proportion is 5-3-2, i.e. five parts carbohydrates, three parts lipids and two parts proteins, a composition close to that of mother's milk.

It is when our food intake matches this 'golden proportion' that calories are then most efficiently assimilated in the small intestine so that it is easy to put on weight.

On the other hand, all you have to do is change this ideal proportion and the calories are not absorbed as well and the energy from the foods is reduced. Theoretically, the most radical modification conceivable, which would reduce most drastically the calories absorbed, would be to restrict our food intake to a single food group.

In practice, even though this has been tried out in the USA with carbohydrates (the Beverly Hills diet allowed only exotic fruits) or fats (the Eskimo diet), it is hard to eat only sugars or fats and this has serious repercussions for our health. Too much sugar allows diabetes to develop easily and too much fat, apart from our inevitable disgust, would pose a major risk to the cardiovascular system. Furthermore, proteins are essential for life and if the body does not get them it raids its own muscle for them.

If we are to eat from one single food group, the only possibility is proteins: a satisfactory solution as far as taste is concerned, it avoids the risk of clogging up the arteries and by definition it excludes protein deficiency.

When you manage to introduce a diet limited to protein

foods, the body has great difficulty in assimilating the chewed food that it was not programmed to deal with and it cannot use all the calories contained in the food. It finds itself working like a two-speed engine, in a scooter, lawnmower or motor boat, designed to run on a mixture of pure petrol and oil but trying to run on pure petrol. It putters and then stalls, unable to use its fuel.

In the same way, when the body feeds on very high protein foods it restricts itself to taking the proteins it needs to survive and for the vital maintenance of its organs (muscles, blood cells, skin, hair, nails) and it makes poor and scant use of the other calories provided.

Assimilating proteins burns up a lot of calories

To understand the second property of protein, which makes the Dukan Diet so effective, you need to familiarize yourself with the idea of SDA, or Specific Dynamic Action, of foods. SDA represents the effort or energy that the body has to use to break down food until it is reduced to its basic unit, which is the only form in which it can enter the bloodstream. How much work this involves depends on the food's consistency and molecular structure.

When you eat 100 calories of white sugar, a quick carbohydrate par excellence composed of simple, barely aggregated molecules, it is assimilated very quickly. The work to absorb it burns up only seven calories, so 93 usable calories remain. The SDA for carbohydrates is seven per cent.

When you eat 100 calories of butter or oil, assimilating

them is a bit more laborious: 12 calories are burned up, leaving only 88 for the body. The SDA of lipids is 12 per cent.

Finally, to assimilate 100 calories of pure protein – egg whites, lean fish, or non-fat cottage cheese – the task is enormous. This is because protein is composed of an aggregate of very long chains of molecules, whose basic links, amino acids, are connected to each other by a strong bond that requires a lot more work to be broken down. It takes 30 calories just to assimilate the proteins, leaving only 70 for the body, i.e. the SDA is now 30 per cent.

Assimilating proteins makes the body work hard and is responsible for producing heat and raising our body temperature, which is why swimming in cold water after eating a protein-rich meal is inadvisable as the change in temperature can result in immersion hypothermia.

This characteristic of proteins, annoying for anyone desperate for a swim, is a blessing for overweight people who are usually so good at absorbing calories. It means they can save calories painlessly and eat more comfortably without any immediate penalty.

At the end of the day, after eating 1,500 calories worth of proteins, a substantial intake, only 1,050 calories remain after digestion. This is one of the Dukan Diet's keys and one of the reasons why it is so effective. But that's not all . . .

Pure proteins reduce your appetite
Eating sweet foods or fats, easily digested and assimilated, does create a superficial feeling of satiety, all too soon

swept away by the return of hunger. Recent studies have proved that snacking on sweet or fatty foods does not delay your urge to eat again, or reduce the quantities eaten at the next meal. On the other hand, snacking on proteins does delay your urge for your next meal and does reduce the amount that you then eat. What is more, if you only eat protein foods this produces ketonic cells, powerful natural appetite suppressants that are responsible for a lasting feeling of satiety. After two or three days on a pure protein diet, hunger disappears completely and you can follow the Dukan Diet without the natural threat that weighs down on most other diets: hunger.

Pure proteins fight oedema and water retention
Certain diets or foods are known as being 'hydrophilic', that is, they encourage water retention and the swelling this causes. This is the case for mostly vegetable diets, rich in fruits, vegetables and mineral salts. Protein-rich diets are the exact opposite. They are known as being water-repellent, in that they promote elimination through urine and, as such, provide a welcome purge or 'drying-out' for tissues gorged with water, which is a particular problem during the premenstrual cycle or during the premenopause.

The Attack diet, made up exclusively of proteins that are as pure as possible, is of all diets the one that best gets rid of water.

This is particularly advantageous for women. When a man gains weight, this is mostly because he overeats and stores his surplus calories in the form of fat. For a woman, how she puts on weight is often more complex and bound up with water retention, which prevents diets from working properly.

At a certain time during the menstrual cycle, in the four or five days before a period starts, or at certain key times in a woman's life, such as puberty, the interminable premenopause or even in the prime of her sexual life if she has hormonal disorders, women, and especially those who are overweight, begin to retain water and start to feel spongy, swollen and puffy-faced in the morning. They are unable to remove rings from their swollen fingers; their legs feel heavy and their ankles swell. With this retention they put on weight; usually this is reversible but it can become chronic.

Even women who diet in order to slim down and avoid this swelling are surprised to find that during these periods of hormonal surge all the little things that worked before no longer have any effect. In all these cases, which are not so rare, pure proteins such as are found in my programme's Attack diet have a decisive and immediate effect. In a few days, sometimes even in a matter of hours, water-soaked tissues begin to dry up, leaving a feeling of wellbeing and lightness that shows up immediately on the scales and greatly boosts motivation.

Pure proteins boost your system's resistance
This is a characteristic well known to nutritionists, which is also more generally recognized. Before tuberculosis

was eradicated through antibiotics, one of the traditional treatments was to overfeed patients by significantly increasing the amount of proteins. At Berck in northern France, one of the top centres for treating tuberculosis, teenagers were even forced to drink animal blood. Today, sports coaches and trainers advocate a protein-rich diet for athletes who demand a lot from their bodies. Doctors give the same advice to increase resistance to infection, for anaemia or to speed up the healing of wounds.

It is advisable to make use of this advantage, because any weight loss, no matter how small, will weaken the body. I have personally seen that the Dukan Diet's Attack phase, composed exclusively of pure proteins, is the most stimulating phase. Some patients have even told me that it had a euphoric effect, both mentally and physically, and that this happened from the end of the second day.

Pure proteins enable you to lose weight without losing muscle or skin tone

There is nothing surprising in this observation when you realize that the skin's elastic tissue, as well as the body's muscular tissue, is made up essentially of proteins. A diet lacking in proteins forces the body to use its own muscles and the skin's proteins, so that the skin loses its elasticity, to say nothing of menopausal women having brittle bones. Combined, these effects cause ageing of the skin, hair and even general appearance which friends and family soon notice, and which can be enough to make you stop the diet early. Conversely, a protein-rich diet and, even more so, a diet made up exclusively of proteins like the Dukan Diet's first diet, has no reason to attack the body's reserves because the body is being given massive protein supplies. Under these conditions, the weight loss is rapid and toning, muscle firmness is maintained and the skin glows, allowing you to lose weight without looking older.

This particular feature of the Dukan Diet might seem of secondary significance to young and curvy women with firm muscles and thick skin, but it is very important for those women approaching their fifties and therefore the menopause or who have less muscle structure or a fine and delicate skin. This is especially important because, and it has to be said here, there are too many women nowadays who manage their figures guided solely by their scales. Weight cannot and should not be the sole issue. Radiant skin, healthy-looking hair, tissue strength and general body tone are criteria that contribute just as much to a woman's appearance.

THIS DIET MUST INCLUDE A LOT OF WATER

The Importance of Drinking Water

The water issue is always a little disconcerting. Opinions and rumours circulate about it, but almost always there is some kind of 'authority' telling you today the exact opposite of what you heard yesterday. However, this water issue is not simply a marketing concept for diets, designed to amuse those who want to lose weight. It is a question of great importance that, despite the enormous combined efforts of the press, doctors, mineral-water manufacturers and simple common sense, has never really totally won over the public and in particular those people on diets.

To simplify things, it may seem essential to burn calories so that our fat reserves melt away; but this combustion, as necessary as it is, is not enough. Losing weight is as much about eliminating as it is about burning.

Would a housewife dream of doing the laundry or washing dishes without rinsing them? It is the same with losing weight and while on this subject it is essential to spell things out. A diet that does not involve drinking a sufficient quantity of water is a bad diet. Not only is it ineffective, but it leads to the accumulation of harmful waste.

Water purifies and improves the diet's results
Simple observation shows us that the more water you drink, the more you urinate and the greater the opportunity for the kidneys to eliminate waste derived from the food burned. Water is, therefore, the best natural diuretic. It is surprising how few people drink enough water.

The many demands in our busy day conspire to delay then finally obliterate our natural feeling of thirst. Days and months go by and the message disappears altogether and no longer plays its part in warning us about tissue dehydration. Many women, whose bladders are smaller and more sensitive than men's, do not drink to avoid having to go to the toilet constantly or because it is awkward at work or on public transport or because they do not like public toilets.

However, what you may get away with under ordinary circumstances has to change when following a weight-loss diet and if healthy lifestyle advice remains unheeded there is one argument that always wins people over:

Trying to lose weight without drinking is not only toxic for the body, but it can reduce and even completely block the weight loss so that all your work is for nothing. Why?

Because the human engine that burns its fat while dieting functions like any combustion engine. Burned energy gives off heat and waste. If these waste products are not regularly eliminated afterwards by the kidneys, they will accumulate and, sooner or later, interrupt combustion and prevent any weight loss, even if you are following the diet scrupulously.

It is just the same for a car engine with a clogged exhaust pipe, or a fire in a fireplace full of ashes. Both end up choking and dying from the build-up of waste. Sooner or later, bad nutrition and the accumulated effects of bad healthcare and extreme or unbalanced diets will make the overweight person's kidneys become lazy. More than anyone else, the overweight person needs large quantities of water to get their excretion organs working again.

At the outset, drinking a lot of water may seem tedious and unpleasant, especially in wintertime. But if you keep it up, the habit will grow on you. Then, encouraged by the pleasant feeling of cleaning out your insides and even better, of losing weight, drinking often ends up once again becoming something you need to do.

When they are combined, water and pure proteins act powerfully on cellulite

This fact only concerns women, as cellulite is a type of fat that, under hormonal influence, accumulates and remains trapped in the most feminine areas of the body: the thighs, hips and knees. Diets are very often powerless against it. I have personally discovered that the pure protein diet, together with a reduction in salt intake and a real increase in consumption of mineral water with a low mineral content, leads to a more harmonious weight loss with moderate but genuine slimming in the difficult areas, such as the thighs or insides of the knees.

Compared to other diets that the patient has followed at different times in her life, this is the combination that for the same amount of weight loss achieves the best overall reduction around the hips and thighs.

These results can be explained by the water-repellent effect of proteins and the intense filtering undertaken by the kidneys made possible by this massive water intake. Water penetrates all tissues, even cellulite. It goes in, pure and clean, and comes out salty and full of waste. Adding the powerful effect of burning up pure proteins to this expulsion of salt and waste brings about definite, even if modest, results. This is a rare achievement and sets the diet apart from most others which have no specific effect on cellulite.

When should you drink water?

People still cling to old wives' tales that would have you believe that it is best not to drink at mealtimes to avoid food trapping the water. Not only does this idea of not drinking at mealtimes have no physiological basis, but in many cases it makes things worse. Not drinking while you eat, at a time when you naturally get thirsty and when drinking is so easy and enjoyable, may result in you suppressing your thirst altogether and then, when you are busy later on with your daily activities, you forget to drink water for the rest of the day. During the Dukan Diet and especially during the alternating proteins phase, except in cases of exceptional water retention caused by hormonal or kidney problems, it is absolutely essential to drink a litre and a half of water a day. If possible drink mineral water or take it in any other liquid form such as tea, herbal tea or coffee.

A cup of tea at breakfast, a large glass of water mid-morning, two more glasses and a coffee at lunch, one glass during the afternoon and two glasses with dinner and you have easily downed a couple of litres. Many patients have told me that in order to drink when they were not thirsty they got into the habit of drinking directly from the bottle and this worked better for them.

Which water should you drink?
- The most suitable waters for the pure protein Attack phase are mineral waters low in sodium, which are slightly diuretic and laxative. Among the best known

are Vittel, Evian, Buxton, Highland Spring, Volvic and Perrier, the famous sparkling variety. You should avoid San Pellegrino and Badoit, which are good but contain too much sodium to be drunk in large quantities.

- If you drink tap water, then continue to do so. It is far more important to drink enough water to get your kidneys working again than it is to worry about what is in the water you are drinking.

- The same holds true for all the various sorts of teas, green teas and herbal teas, which can tempt those people who enjoy their cuppa and, in particular, prefer hot drinks, especially to warm up in winter.

- In the case of diet fizzy drinks, I consider them all to be great allies in the fight against weight problems (or excess weight) as long as they have no more than one calorie per glass. As far as I am concerned not only do I allow them, but I recommend them and for several reasons. First of all, it is often the best way to make sure you drink the one and a half litres of liquid already mentioned. In addition, they have virtually no calories or sugar. Finally, and above all, a fizzy drink like Diet Coke or Coca Cola Zero, the market-leading brand, provides a clever mix of intense flavours, just like traditional Coke, which can reduce the craving for sugar if used repeatedly by those who like snacking on sweet things. Many of my patients have confirmed that diet fizzy drinks were fun and comforting when used as a part of their diet and actually helped them. The sole exception regarding diet fizzy drinks is in the case of a dieting child or teenager. It has been proven that substituting 'fake' sugar does not work and barely reduces their craving for sugar. Furthermore, unlimited use of sweet-tasting fizzy drinks might form a habit of drinking without thirst and just for pleasure, which could make them vulnerable to more dangerous addictions later on in life.

Water is naturally filling

As you know, we often associate the sensation of an empty stomach with being hungry, which is not entirely wrong. Water drunk during a meal and mixed with food increases the total volume of the food mass and stretches the stomach, thereby inducing that feeling of a full stomach, the first signs of satisfaction and satiety: yet another reason for drinking at mealtimes. However, experience proves that keeping the mouth busy works just as well in between meals, for example during the danger zone in your day, between 5 p.m. and 8 p.m. A big glass of any liquid will often be enough to calm your hunger pangs.

Nowadays, the world's richest populations are confronting a new type of hunger: a self-imposed denial of food while surrounded by an infinite variety of foodstuffs, which they dare not touch because of the risk to their health or because they have weight problems.

It is surprising to see that at a time when individuals, institutions and pharmaceutical laboratories dream of discovering the perfect and most effective appetite suppressant, there are so many people for whom this is an issue who still do not know about, or even worse refuse to use, a method as simple, pure and inexpensive as drinking water to tame their appetite.

THE DIET HAS TO BE LOW IN SALT

Kicking the Salt Habit

Salt is an element vital to life and present to varying degrees in any and every food. So adding salt at the table is always superfluous. Salt is just a condiment that improves the flavour of food, sharpens the appetite and is all too often used purely out of habit.

A low-salt diet is never dangerous

You could and even should live your whole life on a low-salt diet. People with heart and kidney problems or high blood pressure live permanently on low-salt diets without suffering harmful effects. However, people with low blood pressure and who are used to living that way should exercise caution.

A diet too low in salt, especially when combined with a large intake of water, can increase the filtering of the blood, washing it out and in doing so even reduce its volume and lower blood pressure further and, if already naturally low, this can produce fatigue and dizziness if you get up quickly. These people should not go overboard with salt reduction and should limit their water intake to one and a half litres per day.

*On the other hand, too much salt leads to water
retention in your body tissue*

In hot climates, salt pills are regularly distributed to workers so that they avoid dehydration from the sun.

For women, especially women intensely influenced by hormones, during premenstrual or premenopausal periods, or even during pregnancy, many parts of the body become spongy, retaining impressive amounts of water.

For these women, this diet, a water-reduction diet par excellence, works most effectively when as little salt as possible is absorbed, allowing the water to pass more quickly through the body, just as it does during cortisone treatment.

By the way, we often hear people complaining that they have put on two or even four pounds in one evening, after a lapse in their diet. Sometimes a weight gain like this is not even due to a real lapse. When we analyze exactly what was eaten, we can never track down the 18,000 calories of food required to produce these four extra pounds. It was simply the combination of an over-salty meal accompanied by drinks; salt and alcohol combine to slow down the throughput of the water drunk. Never forget that one litre of water weighs two pounds and two teaspoons of salt are enough to retain this water in your body's tissues for a day or two.

This being the case, if during your diet you cannot avoid a professional dinner engagement or family celebration that will force you to put aside the rules you are otherwise following, then at least avoid eating salty foods and drinking too much alcohol. And do not weigh yourself the next morning, because a sudden increase in weight may discourage you and undermine your determination and confidence. Wait until the following day, or even better two days, while stepping up the diet, drinking mineral water with a low mineral content and cutting back on salt. These three simple measures should be enough to get you back on track.

Salt increases appetite; decreasing your salt intake decreases your appetite

This is a simple observation. Salty foods increase salivation and gastric acidity, which in turn increase your appetite. Conversely, lightly salted foods have only a slight effect on digestive secretions and no effect on appetite. Unfortunately, the absence of salt reduces thirst and when you follow the Dukan Diet you have to accept that during the first days you will have to make yourself drink a large amount of liquid so that you boost your need for water and re-establish your natural thirst.

Conclusion

The pure protein diet, the initial and principal driving force behind the four integrated diets that make up my programme, is not like other diets. It is the only one to use just a single food group and one well-established category of foods with the highest protein content.

During this diet and throughout the whole programme, any mention of calories and of calorie-counting is to be avoided. Whether a few or many are eaten has little effect on the results. What counts is keeping within this food category. So the actual secret of the programme's first two slimming phases is to eat a lot, even to eat in anticipation, before the hunger pangs take over. Hunger that turns into uncontrollable cravings that can no longer be appeased by the proteins you are allowed to eat leads the careless dieter towards pure comfort foods, foods with little nutritional value, sugary, creamy, rich and destabilizing foods, which nevertheless have a strong emotive power.

The effectiveness of this diet is therefore entirely connected with choosing the right foods, as powerful as lightning when intake is limited to this category of food, but if this rule is not followed it slows right down and you have to resort to miserable calorie-counting. To spell it out, by following this diet you have replaced a calories system with a categories system. There is absolutely no need for you to count calories; all you need do is stay within the categories. But if you stray away from the list of permitted foods, you are no longer allowed to eat any quantity you like and you will have to start counting how many calories you eat.

So this is a diet you cannot follow in half measures. It relies on the great all-or-nothing law which explains not only its metabolic effectiveness, but also its amazing impact on the psychology of an overweight person who also operates according to this same law of extremes.

With a temperament that goes from one extreme to another, just as determined when making an effort and as easy-going when giving up, the overweight person finds in each of the four stages of my programme an approach to suit them perfectly.

These affinities between the individual's psychological profile and the diet's structure create a synergy whose importance is hard for outsiders to understand, but which is decisive for those involved. The mirroring generates a strong bond with the diet that makes losing weight easier but which really comes into its own in the ultimate Stabilization stage. This is when everything rests on the one day of proteins per week, a day of redemption, a measure that is as specific as it is effective; that on its own and in this form can be accepted by anyone who has always struggled with their weight.

THE DUKAN DIET IN PRACTICE

You have now reached the decisive moment of putting my programme into practice. You now know everything you need to understand how it works and the effectiveness of the four diets that make it up. In the introduction to the theory, I also tried to help you understand that people do not become overweight by accident. The pounds you have gained that you now want to get rid of are a part of you that you deny, but a part that is a reflection of your nature, of your psychology and, therefore, of your identity.

This has as much to do with your genes or a family predisposition to put on weight, the way your metabolism works, as your personality, emotions and feelings and, often, your own particular way of using the pleasure from food to deaden life's small and large displeasures.

This goes to show that the problem is not as simple as it seems and explains why so many others, and maybe you too in the past, have failed, why so many diets run out of steam. To struggle against a force as powerful and ancient as the need to eat, an almost animal force that comes from deep inside, is uncontrollable, and which sweeps aside all reasoning, obviously cannot be based simply on rationally learning about nutrition, however thorough this may be, or on the hope that an overweight person will achieve self-control on their own.

To stand any chance against the force of instinct, you have to fight it on its own ground, with means, language and a strategy that come from the same instinctive level. Our need to feel seductive, our need for wellbeing, our fear of illness, our need to belong to a group and conform to prevailing style trends come from this level. Nowadays they are the only instinctive defence forces capable of motivating the overweight. But with the first signs of improvement they fade away; as soon as our self-image improves, our clothes no longer feel too tight or we are able once again to climb stairs without losing our breath, these defences are gone.

But above all, in order for a diet, or better, a comprehensive dieting programme, to stand any chance of being adopted and followed by an overweight person, we need to use another area of instinct: the command of authority. Therefore the recommendation for a programme to slim has to be formulated by an outside authority figure. Another will that takes the place of the overweight person's will and which speaks with precise instructions, which are non-negotiable, not open to interpretation and, above all, are kept in a workable form for as long as you intend to maintain the results. I designed the Dukan Diet based on the remarkable effectiveness of alternating proteins while adjusting the programme over the years to fit the exact particular profile of each patient, creating a whole system of foolproof instructions to channel and make the most of their passionate nature that tends to extremes and their initial heroic efforts, but which would also counterbalance any lapses in their efforts. I also realized that a one-step plan was not adequate for such a complex task. So I devised a programme with four diets, one following the other, a complete and coherent system that never, ever leaves the overweight person to face temptation and failure alone.

Recently I have realized that losing weight without taking exercise, the most simple and natural exercise that there is so that it becomes a part of your long-term routine, runs the risk of undermining this undertaking. In a world where being sedentary is an integral part of our societies' economic model and where it is not only accepted but encouraged, simple common-sense advice is not enough. I have therefore decided to include exercise and in particular walking as a full driving force in my programme. I now no longer just recommend it but I PRESCRIBE it as I would medication. It will be described to you in greater detail in a later chapter.

The Attack Phase: the Pure Protein Diet

However much weight is to be lost over whatever length of time, my programme always starts with the pure protein diet, which is a highly specific diet I use to create a psychological trigger and a metabolic surprise, whose combined effects result in a first decisive weight loss.

I will now review in detail all the foods you will use in

this first phase, adding some advice to the description to make your personal choice easier.

How long does this initial Attack phase have to last in order to achieve its role as trigger and starter? There is no standard reply for this extremely important question. How long it lasts depends on each individual. Above all it depends on how much weight you want to lose, but also on your age, how many previous diets you have tried, how motivated you are and how you feel about proteins.

I will also give you very precise information about the results you can expect from this Attack diet, which obviously rely on it being followed to the letter and for the correct length of time.

Finally, I will outline the various reactions you might encounter during this initial period.

Which Foods Are Allowed?

During this period, which can last from one to ten days, you are allowed to eat foods from the eleven categories on the following list.

From these categories, you can eat as much as you want or suits you, with no limit and at whatever time of day you feel hungry. You may also freely combine foods from any of these categories.

You can just select the ones you like, leaving the others aside, or in extreme cases eat from a single category in one single meal or for one day.

The essential thing is to stick to this precisely defined list. Remember that I have been prescribing it to people for many years and I have not left anything out. You must also realize that succumbing to any other foods, as small as the lapse may be, will be like puncturing a balloon with a needle.

An apparently harmless lapse will be enough for you to lose all the benefits of this precious freedom of being able to eat all you want. For just a tiny gain in quality, you will be forced for the rest of that day to count your calories and restrict what you eat.

In short, the watchword is simple and non-negotiable: you are allowed everything on the following list, with complete freedom. Anything that is not on the list is forbidden, so forget about it for now, knowing that in the near future you will again be eating all the foods that have been removed.

Category 1: Lean meats
By lean meat, I mean two types of meat: veal and beef.

- Beef: all roasts or grilled beef are allowed, namely, steaks, tenderloin, sirloin and roast beef; you must carefully avoid all types of ribs as they are too fatty.
- Veal: recommended are veal escalopes and roast veal; veal cutlets are allowed as long as you trim all the fat.
- Rabbit is a lean meat and can be eaten roasted with mustard or yoghurt.

- Pork and lamb are not allowed in the Attack diet so that it is as effective as possible.

You can prepare all these meats how you like but without using any butter, oil or cream, not even low-fat versions. However, if using a frying pan, you can rub the surface with a few drops of oil on a piece of kitchen paper, to keep the flavour of the cooked meat.

I recommend that you grill your meat, but these meats can also be roasted in the oven, cooked on a rotisserie, or even boiled. How well done or not you like your meat is up to you. But do remember that the longer the meat is cooked, the less fat there is, which comes closest to the Dukan Diet's ideal of pure protein.

Cooked minced meat is recommended for those who may easily grow tired of cuts and who like preparing their meat as burgers or meatballs mixed with an egg, spices, capers or gherkins and cooked in the oven. Raw meat is allowed, *tartare-* or *carpaccio*-style, but it must be prepared without oil. Frozen beefburgers are allowed but make sure that the fat content does not exceed ten per cent – 15 per cent is too rich for the Attack phase. Be careful with kosher burgers, which are very fatty. You would do better to mince some lean meat yourself or cook them so that most of the fat runs off.

I will remind you again that you can eat as much as you want.

Category 2: Offal

Only liver (beef, veal or poultry) and tongue are allowed. Lamb and beef tongue are permitted but only eat the tip of the tongue, which is the leanest part, and avoid the back section which is too fatty. As for liver, it is rich in vitamins, which is very useful during a diet. Unfortunately, it is also high in cholesterol, so should be avoided if you have any cardiovascular problems.

Category 3: Fish

There is no restriction or limitation with this family of foods. All fish are allowed, lean or fat, white or oily, fresh, frozen, dried or smoked, or canned (but not in any oil or sauce containing fat).

- All fatty fish and oily fish are allowed, i.e. sardines, mackerel, tuna and salmon.
- All white and lean fish are also allowed, such as sole, hake, cod, bream, red mullet, catfish, whiting, skate, trout, plaice, monkfish, coley, pollock and sea bass, as well as many other lesser-known varieties.
- Smoked fish is permitted, too; smoked salmon, although greasy-looking, is less fatty than a 90 per cent fat-free steak. The same goes for smoked trout, eel and haddock.
- Canned fish, very handy for quick meals or picnics, is allowed if it is in brine or water like tuna, salmon, mackerel or sardines in tomato sauce.
- Finally, you are allowed to have surimi. Originally from Japan, these crab sticks are made with very lean white

fish and flavoured with crab sauce and a little sugar. Many of my readers have an unfavourable opinion of them. It is true that this is reconstituted food but having researched into how they are produced, I have seen that they are of high nutritional quality, prepared from small white fish on factory ships on the open sea. Others have pointed out to me that the labels mention carbohydrates. This is true but does not rule them out as it is starch, which can be tolerated because of their other qualities. The fat content is in fact very low and crab sticks are extremely practical, odourless and easy to carry around with you.

Always cook your fish without oil or butter, but moisten with lemon or soy sauce, and sprinkle with herbs and spices. Enjoy it baked, poached or steamed.

Category 4: Shellfish
Here I include crustaceans and all shellfish.

- Pink and grey shrimps, Mediterranean prawns, crayfish, crab, winkles, lobster, langoustines, scallops, oysters, clams and mussels.

Keep these in mind and use them to add a festive touch to your menu and make it interesting and varied. They are also very filling and satisfying.

Category 5: Poultry

- All poultry is allowed except birds with flat beaks, such as farm-reared goose and duck, provided you do not eat the skin. Take care to leave the skin on when cooking and remove it on your plate at the last moment so that the meat does not dry out.
- Chicken is the most popular poultry product and the most practical one for the pure protein Attack diet. Everything is allowed except the outside part of the wings, which is too fatty and cannot be separated from the skin. However, you should be aware that different parts of the chicken have differing amounts of fat. The leanest part is the white breast meat, followed by the thigh, then the wing. Finally, the chicken should be as young as possible.
- Turkey in all forms is allowed; turkey breast cooked in a pan, or roast turkey stuffed with garlic. Partridge, guinea fowl and quail are all permitted as well as pheasant and wild duck, which is lean.

Category 6: Low-fat, lean ham, with any rind cut off

For some time now low-fat ham and smoked turkey or chicken have been available in supermarkets. They have a fat content between two and four per cent. This is far below both lean meats and the leanest of fish. They are highly recommended and are very easy to use.

In odourless plastic packs, generally pre-sliced and with no waste, they are perfect to take with you for lunch.

Moreover, even if they do not taste as good as fresh cold meats, their nutritional value is in every respect comparable.

The same goes for thinly sliced dried beef and the Italian version, bresaola, which comes from dried beef fillet. These are very lean and tasty delicatessen products which unfortunately are also relatively expensive. You can find them in packs in supermarkets but they are less salty and more flavoursome if bought from a deli.

Remember that deli hams and cured hams are not allowed; nor is smoked ham, which is even fattier.

Category 7: Eggs

Eggs can be eaten hard-boiled, soft-boiled, poached, or in an omelette, but always without any butter or oil.

To make your eggs more sophisticated and less monotonous, you can add prawns or even some shredded crab. Try omelettes with chopped onion just for the flavour, ham and spices. In a diet where quantities are not restricted, eggs can be problematic because of the cholesterol they contain. Eggs are high in cholesterol and excessive consumption should be avoided by anyone with a high cholesterol level in their blood; in such cases no more than three or four egg yolks should be eaten per week. But the egg white, a pure protein par excellence, can be eaten without restriction. You can make omelettes using just one yolk for every two whites. Some people are allergic to egg yolks but they are usually aware of this and therefore avoid them.

A more frequent problem is indigestion caused by eggs, which is wrongly attributed to a fragile liver. Apart from eggs that are of poor quality or too old, it is not the eggs themselves the liver has difficulty with but the butter used to cook them.

So, if you are not allergic to eggs, do not have a high cholesterol count and you cook them without oil or butter, you may eat two eggs every day without running any risk during this brief Dukan Diet Attack period.

Category 8: Plant proteins

Over the last ten years or so we have witnessed a declining appetite for meat, in particular amongst women. This is the reason why I have introduced this extra category and made it a long and detailed one, so as to find a way round this disenchantment with meat. Plant proteins are proteins produced from soya and wheat. Most of them have come to us from Asia, and in particular from Japan, and so they have benefitted from the current enthusiasm in the West for Japanese food and cooking.

In this eighth category, I've grouped together seven foods that are very high in proteins, but low in fat. However, only the first two, tofu and seitan, which are two foodstuffs produced respectively from soya and wheat, have a sufficient concentration of protein that you may eat them 'as much as you like' as with the previous seven categories.

The five other foods – tempeh, veggie burgers and soya steaks, textured soya protein (TSP), soya milk and soya yoghurt – are very useful foodstuffs, but ones that I am reserving for those vegetarian readers who don't eat meat or fish. For non-vegetarians, these five foods can be used as Tolerated Foods i.e. you may eat only a certain weighed quantity and at certain intervals.

1. Tofu

It is simple and easy to make your own tofu. You crush soya beans in water to produce soya milk and then add salt to coagulate it and produce firm tofu, which has the same texture as feta cheese. To make silken tofu, all you have to do is add a coagulant called 'Nigari' and heat the mixture. You'll find information for these two recipes on loads of cookery websites. For those of you who would prefer not to start from scratch every morning, tofu is now sold by all major retailers and in organic stores.

There are two types of tofu: silken and firm:

- Silken tofu is a cooking ingredient with the consistency of thick custard or yoghurt. It is sold in containers at room temperature, but is best kept for up to three to four days in the fridge. It is particularly useful when making pâtisserie and dessert recipes, and quiches with an oat bran galette base. It is also very handy for sauces, where it can be used to replace mayonnaise or crème fraîche. Because of its texture, it can be whipped and is a worthy rival to whipped cream.
- Regular tofu has the consistency of firm feta cheese and is an ingredient used in many different recipes.

It can be eaten crumbled, grated, diced or mashed and used for all types of main courses, starters and puddings. It is naturally bland, but it soaks up all the flavours of the foods around it. It goes very well with chives, soy sauce and mild spices. You can use it diced in mixed salads or in vegetable flans made with oat bran. Tofu benefits greatly from being marinated in a sauce of your choice for a few hours before you cook with it. Try pressing it between two chopping boards or plates of medium weight as this will squeeze all the water out of the tofu so that it really absorbs all the flavours of your marinade. Firm tofu can be stored like mozzarella – in the fridge and in water, which should be changed every two days and kept no longer than 10 days in total.

In a similar way to crab sticks (surimi), tofu is fast becoming firmly established as a common foodstuff in the West, and it now has a special place in my method. You can find different sorts of prepared tofu: tofu with herbs, curry-flavoured and smoked tofu. And there are even recipes for dishes such as Provence-style tofu, tofu with garlic and herbs, with curry and poppy seeds or with saffron. You can also find substitute tofu veggie sausages, vegetable stir-fries and raviolis – they are all very high quality and surprisingly delicious. However, you need to take care here! None of these dishes and forms of tofu have been prepared following our dietary codes, so you'll need to read the label very carefully to avoid anything with a fat content that exceeds 8 per cent.

2. Seitan

Seitan, or 'vegetable meat', is the equivalent of tofu, but made from wheat protein instead of soya protein. Its resistant texture is like that of meat, so it is often used in stews, hotpots and casseroles. But it can also be cooked as kebabs or in a fricassee or stir-fry. You can buy it ready-made, plain or flavoured, from Asian or organic food stores, and it is sold in blocks, strips and shaped forms.

Since it is simple and cheap to make at home, it is quite possible to make seitan yourself when you have time – and this can be fun too. It is made by washing wheat flour in a fabric bag so that you get rid of all the starch and keep only the gluten. If you don't have much time, you can buy it ready prepared, but then use the time you have saved to cook it skilfully.

Seitan started life as an organic product and one that vegetarians can make use of. I think that it is time to make it available to a wider public and especially to anyone seeking to lose weight while widening the range of foodstuffs they are able to choose from. And in particular, I have in mind those people who are following my method where the first two phases focus so strongly on high-protein and low-fat foods.

As far as nutritional composition is concerned, seitan is extremely high in proteins (25 per cent), low in calories (110 calories per 100g/3½oz) and it contains very little carbohydrate, virtually no fat, no cholesterol or purines.

Seitan may be stored in the fridge for three to four

days (in its stock mix) and for months in the freezer (you can also use it to make vegetable 'mince').

Seitan can be cooked in many ways, however the best way of cooking it is by frying it gently, while the best way to preserve its consistency and flavour is to avoid slicing it too thickly. Why not try marinating it in a mix of soy sauce, herbs, spices and garlic before you fry it. Let the seitan slices soak up the sauce of your choice and then serve it with or without vegetables depending on whether you are in the Attack or Cruise phase. There are lots of great seitan recipes on the internet, such as seitan goulash and seitan kebabs.

3. Tempeh

Tempeh is another foodstuff made from soya. It originally came from Indonesia and is produced by fermenting soya beans. Tempeh has a firm texture and a natural flavour of hazelnut and mushrooms. It's a great food for vegetarians given that it contains lots of protein, little fat and no cholesterol. However, unfortunately tempeh has too much carbohydrate to be fully used in my diet, where it can only feature as a Tolerated Food and not as an 'as much as you like' ingredient.

4. Veggie Burgers and Soya Steaks

These burgers and steaks offer a vegetable alternative to meat and are useful primarily for vegetarians. Usually, meat lovers do not find them totally satisfying and only give them a go if they really have to. However, vegetarians often genuinely like them, especially once they've grown used to them and know how to cook them properly.

Some veggie burgers are soya-based, others are cereal-based and others are essentially vegetable-based. Such diversity impacts greatly on the food's nutritional composition. It is therefore important that you look at the label to check the respective carbohydrate content, which is the limiting factor in my diet.

You must also read the labels carefully for soya steaks because the lipid and fat content can range greatly and one brand can be twice as high as another. Soya steaks can have as low as an eight per cent fat content, which is more or less that of a semi-lean steak you'd buy from your butcher.

5. Textured Soya Protein (TSP)

Textured soya protein looks like tiny granular pebbles similar to praline. TSP is made from defatted soya flour. The flour is mixed with water and heated under pressure. The mixture is then dried and turned into granules, flakes or larger pieces.

TSP offers many advantages as it contains twice as much protein as beef. It is low in calories and has no cholesterol. Easy to store, it can be kept for a very long time. Lastly, TSP is very cheap and easy to cook with. Once cooked, it develops a texture similar to that of meat, which means that vegetarians can enjoy dishes and recipes that are traditionally reserved for meat eaters.

Furthermore, uncooked it has a crunchy consistency and a natural, slightly peanut taste. This makes it a pleasant snacking food, especially for my diet that often cannot offer that sensation of being able to crunch on something crispy.

But don't get carried away! As with tempeh, TSP contains too much carbohydrate, so for my diet it cannot be eaten 'as much as you like', but only as one of your Tolerated Foods.

6. Soya Milk

Soya milk is a non-dairy drink, high in plant proteins, low in calories, with little fat, calcium or vitamin D and no cholesterol. For vegetarians and anyone who is unable to drink cow's milk, has an aversion to its taste, cholesterol issues or is lactose intolerant, soya milk can replace dairy milk. It comes both plain and flavoured and can be used to make any sauce that uses milk, such as béchamel.

Soya milk can be kept for five to seven days in the fridge.

Once again, please take note! Soya milk cannot be eaten 'as much as you like' as part of my diet, but should be limited to two glasses a day to replace skimmed cow's milk – and you must opt for the plain version.

7. Soya Yoghurt

Made from soya milk, soya yoghurt shares the same characteristics and offers an alternative to anyone who is lactose intolerant or has difficulty digesting dairy products and, of course, it is great for pure vegans.

As far as calories and nutrition go, soya yoghurt is hardly any different from yoghurt made from semi-skimmed milk since, depending on the brand, it has an average fat content of two per cent and is cholesterol-free.

Just as with soya milk, soya yoghurt is not allowed to be eaten 'as much as you like' in my diet, but must be limited to two yoghurts a day and, of course, you'll have to stick to plain yoghurt!

Category 9: Non-fat dairy products
(0% fat yoghurt, fromage frais or quark, cottage cheese)
These foods were developed to make losing weight easier. They are real dairy products, just like standard yoghurt and cottage cheese, but without the fat. Just as the transformation of milk into cheese is responsible for the elimination of lactose, the only sugar found in milk, these fat-free dairy products contain practically nothing but protein, which is why they are so useful when we are looking for pure proteins during the Attack phase.

For some years now, milk producers have sold a new generation of yoghurts sweetened with aspartame or enriched with fruit pulp. While aspartame and other flavourings have no calorie content and are just there to make the yoghurts taste better, the added fruit introduces unwanted carbohydrates. This drawback is compensated for by the fact that these gratifying treats give you the opportunity to enjoy a pudding and so can help you follow the overall diet programme. So that the instruction is clear, there are three sorts of 0% fat yoghurt: natural yoghurt, flavoured yoghurts (e.g. coconut, vanilla, lemon), and fruit yoghurts, i.e. with little bits of fruit or a fruit purée base.

- Natural and flavoured yoghurts are both allowed without any restriction.
- Non-fat fruit yoghurts are allowed too but a maximum of two per day. However, if you want a lightning fast start to your Attack phase diet you are better off avoiding them altogether and even more so if you are going through a period when your weight is stagnating.

Category 10: One and a half litres of water per day
This is the only mandatory category on this list. Everything else is optional and you can choose. As I have already told you, and at the risk of repeating myself, drinking this amount of water is indispensable and non-negotiable. Even if you are following the diet very carefully, if you do not thoroughly flush out your system your weight loss will stop. The waste from your burning of fats will accumulate and extinguish the fire.

All types of water are allowed, including spring waters that are slightly diuretic as long as they do not contain too much sodium. If you do not like plain water, you can drink carbonated water, since carbonation has no effect on weight – it is only salt that must be avoided.

In addition, if you do not care for cold drinks, remember that tea, herbal tea, coffee or any other hot drink are all assimilated as water and count towards your obligatory one and a half litres per day.

Finally, diet drinks, such as Diet Coke or any other brand that does not have more than one calorie per glass, are all allowed at every stage of the Dukan Diet. Nutritionists are divided when it comes to drinks sweetened with aspartame. Some think that the body detects and compensates for their trickery whereas others think that their use provokes further cravings for sugar.

As far as I am concerned, my experience has taught me that abstaining from sugar, no matter for how long, never gets rid of the taste or the longing for sugar. So I see no reason to deprive yourself of this calorie-free treat. Furthermore, I have noticed that using these drinks makes following the diet a lot easier and that their sweet flavour, strong smell, colour, bubbles, as well as their association with festivities and fun, all contribute to a powerful sensory gratification that soothes those cravings for 'something else' that so often tempt those of us who like to snack.

This is the moment to talk about the controversy surrounding aspartame. To put it bluntly, it is said to be carcinogenic and I can understand why this is worrying. In my opinion, there is no need for all this controversy. Aspartame has been used as a sweetener by billions of individuals in every country in the world for more than 35 years without ever having given rise to any complaints or side effects and certainly not any human cancers. As far as I am concerned, and even more importantly as far as the European and world authorities are concerned, I see no reason at all to deprive people on a diet who particularly like sweet tastes. Denying them sweet tastes is certainly not going to make their longing for sweet things disappear. Forbidding them sweet tastes only creates frustration which sooner or later exacts revenge.

Category 11: One and a half tablespoons of oat bran
For years, the first two actual slimming phases in my programme did not contain any starchy foods, any cereals or any flour-based foods. The programme worked fine without them but many of the men and women who followed it eventually ended up longing for carbohydrates.

I discovered oat bran while attending a cardiology conference in America, where there was a presentation on how it reduces cholesterol and diabetes. I brought some home and one morning, having run out of flour, I created a special pancake, which I now call the Dukan oat bran galette, for my daughter, Maya. It is made of oat bran, an egg and some fromage frais or quark, sweetened with aspartame. As she loved it and felt completely full, this spurred me on to suggest to my patients that they try the galette. Their enthusiasm for it persuaded me to include it in my method and my books. This is how oat bran gradually became a fundamental part of my method, the only carbohydrate allowed among the proteins and even within the sanctuary of the Attack phase. Why?

Firstly, from a clinical perspective I very quickly noticed an improvement in results: my patients followed the diet better over the long term; they felt less hungry and full sooner; and all in all were much less frustrated.

I tried to understand how oat bran works and looked at the studies available on it. Oat bran is the fibrous husk that surrounds and protects the oat grain. The grain, used to make rolled oats, is rich in simple sugars. Oat bran is the grain's jacket with few simple sugars but very rich in proteins and particularly in soluble fibres. These fibres have two physical properties which give oat bran its medicinal role.

Firstly, there is its ability to absorb – it can absorb up to 20 times on average its volume of water. This means that as soon as it reaches the stomach, it swells and takes up enough space to make you very quickly feel full. It is also extremely viscous. Once in the small intestine along with food that has by now turned into a pulp, it starts to behave like flypaper and all the surrounding nutrients stick to it. It stops them being absorbed into the blood and it takes some away with it into the stools.

As oat bran makes you feel full up and lose calories, it is a precious ally in my battle against the weight problem epidemic. I say my battle because using oat bran does not take away one of the main advantages my method offers: unlimited access to my 100 foods which you can eat as often and AS MUCH of as you like. Low-calorie diets obviously cannot derive so much benefit from oat bran as they already include starchy foods and even some sugary foods weighed out in limited quantities.

I have done some work of my own to check how oat fibres work. Using coprological studies we can compare the calorie content of the stools of individuals when they have eaten oat bran and when they have not. From this I could see that the brans available were not all as good as each other; and the way bran is produced greatly determines how effective it is. Canada and Finland are the main countries to produce oat bran. I have had the opportunity to work with Finnish agricultural engineers and discovered that two manufacturing parameters, milling and sifting, turned out to be crucial. Milling involves grinding the bran and determines the size of its particles; sifting involves separating the bran from the oat flour.

If the milling is too fine this sterilizes the bran and it loses almost all its effectiveness. Likewise if the bran is too coarse and has not been ground enough its useful surface viscosity is lost. If the bran is not thoroughly sifted it is not sufficiently pure and contains too much flour. However, really thorough sifting makes it too expensive. Working with agricultural engineers and the coprological study of stools, we worked out an effectiveness index for bran to cover milling and sifting which allows its best medicinal effects to develop.

Milling should ideally produce particles with a medium+ size (technically called M2bis). As for sifting, it is after it has been sifted for a sixth time, B6, that oat bran has negligible fast carbohydrate content. These two indexes together make up the overall M2bis-B6 index.

Most manufacturers, and Anglo-Saxon manufacturers in particular, only sell bran to be used in cooking, in porridge for example, which is a real national institution in Britain. They prefer bran to be milled very finely and are not that bothered about the sifting as long as the bran tastes soft and creamy, but its medicinal effects are compromised. The recommended type of bran can be found on our website www.thedukandiet.co.uk.

During the Attack phase, I prescribe a dose of one and a half tablespoons of oat bran per day. I recommend eating it as a savoury galette or sweetened with aspartame and prepared as follows:

The Dukan Oat Bran Galette

Put $1\frac{1}{2}$ tablespoons of oat bran in a bowl, add $1\frac{1}{2}$ tablespoons of non-fat fromage frais or quark and one egg white, or a whole egg if you do not have any cholesterol problems. Sweeten with 1 tablespoon of aspartame or add a little salt according to your taste. Mix all the ingredients thoroughly and pour on to a non-stick pan that has been greased beforehand with a few drops of oil then wiped with kitchen paper. Cook for 2–3 minutes on each side.

The galettes keep for at least a week in the fridge, but wrap them in foil or clingfilm so that they do not dry out. You can also freeze them as they will not lose their taste, texture or nutritional value.

Most of my patients eat their galette first thing, so that they avoid feeling famished mid-morning. Others eat them for lunch with a nice slice of smoked salmon or some thinly sliced dried beef. Other patients have them late afternoon, at the 'danger hour' when cravings can overtake them. Or even after supper when they want to rummage around in cupboards to find a final treat before bedtime.

It should be noted that oat bran galettes are a fantastic weapon against bulimia. My slimming programme is of course not for bulimia sufferers but there may be some who read this book and I know from using oat bran regularly with my patients that it can help them greatly and that they can prepare as many galettes as they want, however they want with the flavours they like, and that this will help them avoid their worst crises when they can consume huge amounts of calories from very poor quality food.

But even if a person is not bulimic, it is possible to go through difficult periods when irrepressible cravings can put paid to a carefully designed and structured slimming phase. In such unusual circumstances, for a day or two (and I really do mean for a day or two) you can eat more oat bran and up to three galettes per day.

Extras

Skimmed milk, either fresh, in cartons or powdered, is allowed and can improve the taste and the consistency of tea or coffee; it can also be used to make sauces, cream desserts, custard tarts and many other dishes.

Sugar is not allowed, but aspartame, the best known and most widely used sweetener in the world, is perfectly acceptable and can be used without restriction, even by pregnant women, which proves just how harmless it is.

Vinegar, spices, herbs, thyme, garlic, parsley, onion, shallots, etc. are not only allowed but highly recommended. Using them brings out the flavour of foods and heightens their sensory value. These oral sensations trigger our nervous system which is responsible for whether we feel full or not, contributing to our feeling of being satisfied. To be clear, I am saying quite simply that spices are not just taste enhancers, which in itself is no small achievement, but that they are foods that encourage weight loss. What certain spices such as vanilla or cinnamon do is offer their warm and reassuring taste in exchange for sugary flavours. Others such as coriander, curry powder, colombo (Caribbean curry spice) powder and cloves can cut down the need for salt, especially for women who suffer from water retention who want to add salt to everything before they have even tasted it.

Gherkins, as well as pickled onions, are allowed as long as they are condiments. If eaten in too large a quantity they become a vegetable and outside the Attack phase's pure protein requirement.

Lemons can be used to flavour fish or seafood, but cannot be consumed as lemon juice or lemonade, even without sugar, because although sour, lemons are still a source of sugar and are therefore incompatible with the programme's first two phases, the Attack and Cruise phases.

Mustard and salt are acceptable but must be used in moderation. This is particularly true when it comes to water retention, common among teenage girls whose periods are irregular and in premenopausal women or women following hormone treatment. There are salt-free mustards and low-sodium diet salts if you want to use them liberally.

Ordinary ketchup is not allowed because it is both very salty and very sweet, but there are sugar-free natural ketchups that can be used in moderation and there are high-quality tomato purées such as the famous Heinz varieties that turn into a real treat with just a little flavouring and spicing up – without any of that sweet after-taste, which does not go well with meats.

Chewing gum deserves better than this single entry in the extras category. To my mind it is extremely useful in the fight against weight problems and especially so during my programme's first two slimming phases, the Attack and Cruise phases. I do not usually eat gum myself as chewing is not elegant, but if I am overstressed I do have some then. 'Bruxism' is what dentists call the night-time habit of grinding your teeth until the enamel is worn down. And as a lot of overweight people often eat 'under stress', chewing gum can slow down this mechanical swing towards eating whenever you feel under pressure. What is more, a mouth that is busy chewing gum cannot take or chew anything else so this is a technique for keeping your mouth full. Moreover, there are some sugar-free chewing gums that are absolutely delicious and packed with different flavours, sometimes intense and stimulating flavours. Many scientific studies have also proved at regular intervals how useful chewing gum is when battling against weight problems, diabetes and even tooth decay.

What should we think about the nutritional content of sugar-free chewing gum and which ones should we choose? Of course we are only talking here about so-called sugar-free gum. What this means is that there is no white table sugar or sucrose but the sweeteners used are still sugars and contain almost as many calories as the white variety. Fortunately their ability to sweeten is hundreds of times more powerful than that of ordinary sugar; they are absorbed in the stomach and assimilated very slowly indeed and they have very little effect on insulin and fat storage. Select your sugar-free chewing gum according to taste but go for the ones whose flavour lasts longest in your mouth.

All oil is forbidden. Even though olive oil justifiably has a reputation for protecting the heart and arteries, it is still oil and pure lipids have no place in a pure protein diet.

Shirataki is a new addition to my diet and is unlimited starting from Attack phase. The konjac root from Asia (China and Japan) is satisfying, rich in fibre, stimulates intestinal transit and has virtually no calories. You can use any form of konjac for Dukan cooking, including the noodles, rice, pasta, 'flour' and gel.

Apart from these extras and the eleven major food categories just described, you may eat NOTHING ELSE.

All the rest, anything that is not explicitly mentioned on this list, is forbidden during the Attack diet's relatively brief kick-start period.

Concentrate on what you are allowed to eat and forget the rest. Make sure you get enough variety and pick ingredients for your meals in any order you want so as to keep things interesting. And do not ever forget that all the foods allowed and on this list are for you, really and truly for you.

Some General Advice

Eat as often as you like
Do not forget that the secret of this diet is to eat a lot and to eat before hunger strikes so that you avoid succumbing to a tempting food not on the list.

Never skip meals
This is a bad mistake that often stems from good intentions but which can, little by little, destabilize your diet. Whatever you save by not eating one meal you not only make up for by eating more at the next, but your body reverses this initial economy by increasing the 'profit' it gets out of the next meal, by extracting every last calorie. Furthermore, if you suppress and fuel your hunger, you will be driven towards more comforting foods, forcing you to rely increasingly on your willpower to resist and eventually the strain will undermine even your best intentions.

Drink whenever you eat

For some strange reason, an outdated piece of advice from the 1970s not to drink at mealtimes still remains in the public mind. This idea holds no interest for ordinary mortals and can be harmful for those on a diet, particularly a pure protein diet, because not drinking at mealtimes may make you forget to drink at all. Drinking at mealtimes also increases gastric volume and makes you feel full and satisfied. Finally, water dilutes food and slows down its absorption so that you feel satiated for longer.

Do not run out of the foods you need for your diet

Always have to hand or in your fridge a wide choice of the nine food categories that are going to become your best friends and favourite foods. Take them with you whenever you go out because, unlike lipids and carbohydrates, most protein foods require some preparation and they do not keep as long as, say, biscuits or chocolate in a cupboard or drawer.

Before you eat something, check it is on the list

Just to be extra sure, keep this list with you during the first week. It is simple and can be summed up in a few words: lean meats, offal, poultry, lean ham, all fish and seafood, eggs, plant proteins, non-fat dairy products and water.

Breakfast

Breakfast is an important meal in our pure protein diet. Coffee or tea, sweetened with aspartame if you like, with or without skimmed milk, and enjoyed with a non-fat yoghurt, boiled egg, a slice of turkey or light ham is much better nutritionally than a pastry or chocolate-flavoured cereal, and it is also more satisfying and stimulating.

Breakfast is the perfect time to cook your oat bran galette (see page 76). If you are in too much of a hurry to make the galette, you can eat the oat bran as porridge by mixing a tablespoonful of bran with some hot milk sweetened with aspartame, or mix it with yoghurt to give it a cereal taste and a thicker texture. Take care! During this Attack phase you must not exceed the daily dose of one and a half tablespoons of oat bran so as not to disrupt the specific action of the proteins.

Eating in restaurants

With a little imagination, the pure protein diet is easy to follow. Fish, seafood, poultry and meat generally come in many different guises. You should be able to find some that have been prepared without any fat. You may have to ask to have your dish without the sauce. The difficulty comes afterwards when pudding fans are tempted to eat something sweet. The best strategy is to have a coffee, or you may find that some restaurants now serve low-fat dairy products. Otherwise you can always have a non-fat yoghurt or fruit yoghurt in your car or at the office so that you can end your meal on a satisfying note.

How Long Should the Attack Diet Last?

A decisive choice

This is one of the most important decisions in the Dukan Diet, because this pure protein attack is not only the kick-start that gives you the initial impetus, but it also moulds and sets the tone for the programme on which the three other diets will be based until your permanent stabilization.

Proteins are extremely dense foods that remain present for a long time in the digestive system, making us feel full. As they disintegrate during metabolism, ketone bodies are produced which are well known for creating a feeling of satiety. These two properties mean that proteins are great for combating compulsive behaviour and introducing order into unbalanced eating habits. Finally, because it is extremely effective, this diet produces obvious and immediate results so that you feel powerful and enthusiastic, pumping up your motivation for the long-term haul. That is why it is so important to succeed in this first stage and to decide on its exact ideal duration.

On average the Attack diet lasts five days

This is the time the diet needs to produce its best results without encountering resistance from the body's metabolism before the dieter becomes weary of it. This is also the attack period that best suits the sort of weight loss that most people want to achieve, i.e. between 20 and 40 pounds. On pages 89–91 we'll see the results you should achieve if you follow this diet correctly.

For less ambitious weight loss under 20 pounds
A three-day attack best suits this goal as it allows you to proceed effortlessly to the alternating proteins phase.

For a weight loss under ten pounds
If you would rather avoid an all-too-rapid start, a single day may be enough. This first day, the opening day, heralds a new start, takes your body by surprise and produces an astonishing weight loss that is enough to encourage you to get started with the diet programme.

For serious cases of obesity
In very rare cases, when the target is to lose over 40 pounds, when motivation is really intense or when previous experience with other diets has always resulted in the lost weight being regained, this phase may last seven days or even as long as ten days. But only after medical advice has been taken and on the express condition that enough fluids are drunk throughout the entire period.

How the Body Reacts During the Pure Protein Diet

The surprise effect and the need to adapt to a new way of eating
The first day of the Attack diet is one of adaptation and combat. Of course, the door is open to many categories of popular and tasty foods, but it is firmly closed to other categories that the overweight are in the habit of eating without thinking about just how many and the quantities they consume.

If you feel restricted, and this can overwhelm the less motivated, then the best remedy is to take full advantage of this diet: it's the first diet that allows you to eat as much as you want of foods as dense and prized as beef, veal, fish of every kind, including smoked salmon, tinned tuna, haddock, surimi or crab sticks, oysters, prawns, boiled eggs, low-fat ham, fat-free yoghurts and the whole endless variety of non-fat dairy products.

On the first day, eat more than you would normally. Make up for the foods you cannot eat with the quantity of the foods you can have. And, above all, organize yourself so that you always have all these vital foods to hand, available at all times, in your fridge and cupboards.

Also, by drinking more water than you have ever drunk before, you will feel as if 'there is something there' and more satisfied. You will need to go to the loo more often because, not being used to drinking so much, your kidneys will be forced to open their valves and eliminate. This drainage will relieve water-logged tissues, more common in women, particularly in the thighs, legs and ankles, fingers – swollen to trap rings that have become too tight – as well as in the face. The next morning, get on your scales and you will be amazed by your first results.

Weigh yourself frequently, especially during the first three days. From one hour to the next, you could see new results. Get into the habit of weighing yourself every day of your life because, while for those who put on weight the scales are an enemy, they are a friend and just reward for anyone who loses weight and any weight loss, no matter how tiny, will be your very best incentive.

You might feel a little tired during the first two days and not up to prolonged activity
This is the surprise period when your body is burning up calories without counting or resisting, so it is not the right time to push it to extremes. Avoid hard physical exercise, competitive sports and, in particular, skiing at high altitude. If you already do some gentle gymnastics, jogging or swimming keep this up but, whatever you do, make sure you walk for 20 minutes a day as this is an integral part of the programme. As you will see in the chapter on exercise, these 20 minutes are not just recommended they are prescribed and this means they are non-negotiable.

By the third day, your tiredness will disappear, and is usually replaced by a sense of euphoria and dynamic energy further reinforced by the encouraging messages on your scales.

Bad breath and a dry mouth
These symptoms are not just specific to a protein diet but to any weight-loss diet, although they will be more evident here than in more gradual diets. They are a sign that you are losing weight and as such you should welcome them as proof of success. You can ease them by drinking more.

After the fourth day expect some constipation
For those who are already prone to constipation and those who do not drink enough this is even more

likely. For others, bowel movements may simply be less frequent, but do not take this as a sign of constipation. It is just a reduction in the amount of waste due to the low fibre content of proteins and because you are not yet allowed to eat foods that contain the most fibre, such as vegetables and fruit. If this bothers you, buy some wheat bran flakes and add a tablespoonful along with your oat bran to your galette or to your dairy products.

Above all, drink as much as is recommended, because water not only makes you urinate, but it also softens the stools, improving intestinal contractions and digestion. If you suffer from real constipation this is unpleasant and you must do something about it. Your pharmacist can offer advice and may recommend some natural products based on fruit fibres such as prunes. If this is not enough then you need to see your doctor. Try to resist the temptation to take laxatives, which are too aggressive and which you eventually become used to, so although they work temporarily you have to increase the dosage.

Hunger disappears after the third day

If you do not eat any sugar, this surprising disappearance is linked to the increased release of ketonic cells, the most powerful natural hunger-suppressants. For anyone who is not a big fish- and meat-eater, weariness sets in and monotony has a marked effect on their appetite. Hunger pangs and cravings for sugar disappear completely. The quantity of protein consumed, considerable over these first days, gradually decreases.

Should You Take Vitamins?

I do recommend this, but it is hardly compulsory for such a short period of only three to five days. On the other hand, if the Cruise diet has to deal with a major weight problem and is to last some time, it is a good idea to take multivitamins, but do avoid taking too many different ones and mixing them unwisely as this could have a toxic effect. In practice, it is preferable to simply eat foods packed with vitamins or brewer's yeast. As soon as vegetables are allowed, you can have mixed salads with plenty of lettuce, raw peppers, tomatoes, carrots and cucumbers.

What Results Can I Expect from the Attack Diet?

General factors of resistance or facilitation

The weight loss the pure protein diet produces is the most you could hope for in such a short period of time with a diet consisting of real food. It produces the same results as a protein powder diet, or even total fasting, without any of their main drawbacks. Nevertheless, the weight loss depends on how many extra pounds you have at the outset. Obviously, someone who weighs over two hundred pounds is going to shed those first pounds more easily than someone just wanting to lose a few extra pounds before going on holiday.

Some people have also been 'vaccinated' against dieting by their previous failures with other diets. Age is significant too. For women, hormones play such an important role during puberty, after pregnancy, with oral contraception and, I cannot emphasize this too strongly, during the menopause and post-menopause and peaking especially with any temporary or prolonged hormone therapy treatment.

4 - 10 lbs *For a five-day pure protein Attack diet*

This is generally the most popular and most effective time span and usually the weight lost varies between four and seven pounds. It may reach eight or even ten pounds for someone who is very overweight, especially an active man, or, at worst, it may only be a couple of pounds for a menopausal woman on hormones who is prone to water retention and oedema.

You should also be aware that a woman's body retains water for three to four days before her period starts. This retention reduces the elimination of waste and stops the combustion of fat, momentarily reducing the diet's effectiveness and blocking weight loss.

It is important to realize that before a period starts, the weight-loss process has not been interrupted, just camouflaged and delayed by water retention, and that it will resume two or three days after the period. If not properly explained and understood, this premenstrual plateau can make women despair, as they understandably think that all their efforts have been in vain, undermining their determination and prompting them to give the diet up. So please, always wait until the end of your period before taking such a decision, because as soon as you eliminate the water, your low tide after the premenstrual high tide is when you often see the scales go down at a dizzying rate. If you have to get up to go to the loo several times in the course of one night, you might even lose two to four pounds.

If the Attack phase lasts just three days
You can expect to lose between two and five pounds.

For a single, first-day Attack
Often people lose around two pounds because the surprise effect is always greatest on the first day.

Attack Diet Summary

During this period, which can vary between one and ten days depending on your circumstances, you have unlimited access to the food categories listed below.

From these eleven categories you can eat all you want, without any restriction, at whatever time of day. Think of it as an all-day Eat As Much As You Want buffet. You are also free to mix and match these foods.

The watchword is very simple and non-negotiable: you can have everything on the list without exception; everything that is not on the list is banned, so forget about those foods for the moment, knowing that very soon you will have them all again.

1. Lean meats: beef (except ribs and rib eye), veal, grilled or roasted without oil or fat

2. Offal: kidneys, liver, beef tongue (tip)
3. All poultry, except duck and goose, but without the skin
4. All fish, fatty, lean, white, oily, raw or cooked
5. All shellfish
6. Low-fat ham, sliced low-fat chicken and pork
7. Eggs
8. Plant proteins
9. Non-fat dairy products
10. At least one and a half litres of water with a low salt content
11. The oat bran galette or 1½ tablespoons of oat bran added to milk or a dairy product
12. A compulsory 20-minute walk per day
13. Extras: coffee, tea, vinegar, flavourings, spices, herbs, pickles, lemon (not lemonade), salt and mustard (in moderation)

Apart from these extras and the main food categories described, EAT NOTHING ELSE. All the rest, anything and everything that is not expressly mentioned on this list, is forbidden during the relatively brief period of time that the Attack phase lasts.

Therefore, concentrate on everything you are allowed to have and forget the rest. Vary your meals, mix and match in whatever order, make your menus interesting and never forget that you can have as much as you want of all the foods on this list.

The Cruise Phase: the Protein + Vegetable Diet

At the end of the Attack phase, the Dukan Diet is underway and the alternating protein diet begins – the Cruise phase – which will take you straight to your chosen weight.

This phase actually consists of two alternating diets: one day, the protein + vegetable diet, and then the pure protein diet and so on until you reach your target weight.

Having examined in detail how the pure protein Attack diet works, now let's look at the protein + vegetable diet.

Here again, as with the Attack phase, there is not a standard version of the alternating rhythm of the two diets for everyone, but it is adapted to each person and situation based on the factors that I will describe shortly.

For a long time the rhythm I used most frequently was the 5/5 alternating rhythm, five days of proteins + vegetables with five days of pure proteins. With time and especially for people wanting to lose over 20 pounds I have slowly come round to the 1/1 alternating rhythm with a single day of proteins + vegetables followed by a single day of pure proteins. My own statistics showed that at the end of the first month, the weight loss for both groups was the same and this was perfectly understandable since, after 30 days, each group had had 15 days of proteins and 15 days of proteins + vegetables. But more decisively, over the long term, the risk of tiring of the 5/5 alternating rhythm was greater than for the 1/1 one.

Through meeting readers and studying their letters I have observed that the majority have always gone for the most radical solutions, such as seven to ten days of Attack and then the 5/5 alternating rhythm. This confirms one of my most persistent observations as a practitioner: that when an overweight person who has resisted the idea of dieting for a long time feels motivated to suddenly start dieting, they know perfectly well that the force that has suddenly taken them over is as powerful as it is fragile, and that the best way to maintain it is to follow as closely as possible instructions that are as precise, simple, focused, concrete and non-negotiable as possible. For this reason, I am asking you to trust me and to follow this Cruise phase using the 1/1 alternating rhythm.

By the time you finish the protein-only Attack diet, especially after five whole days, you really start to sorely miss one particular food category: vegetables, raw or cooked, which is great because this is just the right time to introduce them.

I will state this clearly: everything that was allowed in the pure protein diet is still allowed, with the same freedom of quantity, time of day and combinations. Just do not make the mistake of eating only vegetables and no proteins.

Vegetables You Can and Cannot Eat

From now on, as well as protein-rich foods, you are allowed all cooked or raw vegetables and, here again, without restriction regarding quantity, time of day or combination.

You can eat tomatoes, cucumbers, radishes, spinach,

asparagus, leeks, green beans, cabbage, mushrooms, celery, fennel and all types of salads, aubergines, courgettes, peppers and even carrots and beetroot, provided you do not have them at every meal.

Vegetables considered to be starchy foods are, however, forbidden: potatoes, rice, corn, fresh or dried peas, beans and lentils. Avocado is also forbidden; it is not a vegetable, but a fruit, and a very fatty, oleaginous fruit into the bargain, although many people eat them, mistaking them for green vegetables. Salsify and Jerusalem artichokes are also banned.

How should these vegetables be prepared?

Raw or cooked. For everyone who can digest raw vegetables, it is always preferable to eat vegetables when they are fresh and uncooked so that you do not lose any of the vitamins they contain.

The Problem with Dressings

They may appear harmless but dressings are a major problem for weight-loss diets. Indeed, many people base their diet around salads and crudités, which are low in calories and rich in fibre and vitamins. This is perfectly true, but do not forget that it is the dressing that upsets the balance of these good qualities. Let's take a simple example: in an ordinary salad bowl containing two heads of lettuce and two tablespoons of oil, the salad accounts for 20 calories and the oil for 280 calories. The calories sneak in craftily, which is why so many diets based on mixed salads fail because they forget to take into account the calories contained in the dressings.

We also need to clear up the ambiguity concerning olive oil. Even though this now legendary oil, symbol of the Mediterranean lifestyle, is recognized as protecting us against cardiovascular disease, it is no less rich in calories than any other oil on the market.

For these reasons, during the first two actual slimming phases, the Attack and Cruise phases, it is crucial that you avoid preparing green vegetables, cooked or raw, with a sauce or dressing that contains more than a teaspoon of vegetable oil.

Vinaigrette

Here is an easy, flavoursome vinaigrette that uses a tiny amount of oil:

Take an old empty mustard jar and put in it:
1 tablespoon mustard, Dijon or even better French Meaux à l'ancienne with its tiny mustard seeds; 5 tablespoons balsamic vinegar; 1 teaspoon vegetable oil; salt and freshly ground black pepper. If you like garlic, add a large clove to marinate in the bottom of the jar, together with 7 or 8 basil leaves.

If you do not like balsamic vinegar that is a pity as it is more appealing to the senses but you can select another one, just use a little less: 4 tablespoons for wine, sherry or raspberry vinegar and 3 for spirit vinegar.

You must understand that vinegar is a condiment that can play a major role in any diet. An interesting paradox has recently been discovered: that man can distinguish four universal flavours – sweet, salty, bitter and sour – yet vinegar is the only substance in man's food list to provide that precious and rare sour taste.

What is more, recent studies have also demonstrated the impact that oral sensation, the quantity and the variety of flavours, has on producing the feeling of satisfaction and fullness. For example, we know today that certain spices, such as cloves, ginger, turmeric, star anise and cardamom, provide extreme flavours. They bring together strong, penetrating sensations that work on the hypothalamus, the area in our brain that measures these sensations until the feeling of satiety is triggered. So it is very important to use as wide a range of spices and as much as possible, preferably at the start of a meal, and if you are not already a great fan to try to get used to them.

Yoghurt dressing

It is also easy to make a savoury sauce with non-fat dairy products. You can even use natural yoghurt if you prefer. It is creamier than non-fat yoghurt and just a touch more calorific. Add a tablespoon of mustard (Dijon, if possible) and beat the mixture together until it has the consistency of mayonnaise. Add a dash of vinegar, and some salt, pepper and herbs.

Vegetables as a Cooked Garnish

Now is your chance to use green beans, spinach, leeks and cabbage of all varieties, mushrooms, braised greens, fennel and celery. These vegetables can be cooked in water, boiled or, even better, steamed, to retain the maximum amount of vitamins. You can also bake them in the oven in the juices from your meat or fish, such as in classic dishes like sea bass with fennel, sea bream with tomatoes or beef-stuffed cabbage.

Finally, cooking 'en papillote' (in aluminium foil) combines all the advantages as far as nutrition and taste are concerned; it is particularly suitable for preparing fish, in particular salmon, which remains tender when cooked on a bed of leeks or aubergines.

Introducing vegetables after the pure protein phase brings freshness and variety to the initial Attack diet. Things are easier, even comfortable. Now it is practical to start a meal off with a salad, well seasoned, rich in colour and flavour; or, in winter, with a soup, followed by a meat or fish dish gently stewed with flavoursome and fragrant vegetables.

How Many Vegetables Are You Allowed?

In principle, quantity is not limited. But it is wise not to go beyond common sense simply to take advantage of the fact that you are not restricted. I know patients who eat huge mixed salads without even feeling hungry, chomping through their meal as if they had a mouth full of chewing gum. Beware of this, because vegetables are not that harmless. Eat until you no longer feel hungry but do not keep going. This does not alter the rule that quantities are unrestricted, which is at the heart of my programme and by extension of my method.

Whatever quantity you eat, you will still lose weight, but at a slower and less encouraging rate.

With regard to this, I want to tell you about a frequent reaction to the changeover from the strictly protein Attack diet to the diet now improved by the introduction of vegetables.

Very often, weight loss is spectacular during the first phase and then, when vegetables are introduced, the scales seem to get stuck and do not go down, or may even show a slight increase in pounds. Do not worry – you are not slipping backwards. So what *is* happening?

During the Attack phase, because you are eating only proteins this has a powerful water-repellent effect. Reserve fat is lost as well as a large quantity of water that had been stagnating in the body for a long time. This combination of eliminated water and fat explains why your scales show an impressive loss.

But when vegetables are added to proteins, water, having been artificially expelled, is retained once more, which explains the sudden and incomprehensible stagnation. The real weight loss, which is connected to the fats still continues, albeit reduced by the addition of vegetables, but it is being camouflaged by the return of water. Be patient, and as soon as the pure protein days return, the great water expulsion will start again and you will see how many pounds you have really lost.

You must realize, however, that this is going to be your way of life during this period of alternating diets, until you reach your target weight. It is always going to be the pure protein days that get the machine moving and that are responsible for the diet's overall effectiveness. So do not be surprised to see your weight go down at regular intervals. The weight loss levels out during the vegetable days and then drops down to another level during the pure protein days, and so on.

Alternating Rhythm

The diet of alternating proteins, building on the momentum and speed generated by the pure protein Attack diet, is now responsible for guiding you to your chosen goal. This stage will occupy the largest part of the strictly weight-loss period of the Dukan Diet.

The rhythmical addition of vegetables greatly reduces the pure proteins' impact and gives this entire second phase in the diet a kind of syncopated pace, both for organizing your meals and for the results obtained. Indeed, weight loss throughout these weeks will concentrate on the pure protein periods when your body has no means of resisting the power of the Attack, but every time vegetables reappear your body resumes control of the situation and is able to resist. So, there will be pauses interrupted by accelerations, a series of conquests followed by resting periods, all leading in alternate sequence, nevertheless, to your end goal.

What rhythm should this diet take?
I have already explained this but I will sum it up briefly.

- In the short term the most effective rhythm is 5/5: five days of pure proteins followed by five days of proteins + vegetables. It is not the easiest one: it does start off spectacularly but it slows down and may become wearisome with all the risks that this involves.

- The other solution is the 1/1 rhythm: one day of pure proteins followed by one of vegetables + proteins. This alternating rhythm takes longer to get going but in 20 days it will have caught up; and over the long term it is easier to follow and generates less frustration.

- There is a third way, which is suitable if you only have a little weight to lose, the 2/7 rhythm: i.e. two days of pure proteins on Mondays and Thursdays and then five days of proteins + vegetables.

- Finally, there is a variation on the 2/7 rhythm – the 2/0, i.e. two days of pure proteins per week, on Mondays and Thursdays, followed by five normal days of no particular diet but avoiding any extremes. This is the diet that best suits some women with cellulite, who are slim on top but heavy around the hips and the thighs especially. This diet, especially if combined with treatment for those specific areas (mesotherapy) together with sufficient doses of *Centella asiatica* (Gotu Kola), gives the best results for problem areas while sparing the upper body as much as possible.

Oat bran

During the Cruise phase, the amount of oat bran you should eat is two tablespoons per day, prepared in the same way as for the Attack phase.

Exercise

A 30-minute walk. If you are on a stagnation plateau increase this to a 60-minute walk for four days, just till you 'break through' this plateau.

How Much Weight Can You Expect to Lose?

For those who are significantly overweight, by 40 pounds or more, the loss is difficult to predict week by week, but experience has shown that one can expect to lose around two pounds a week.

During the first half of the diet, the loss will be greater, between three and four pounds at the start, which means you can lose the first 20 pounds in approximately two months.

Beyond the first two months, the curve decreases progressively because of a metabolic defence mechanism that I will explain in further detail when we come to the Consolidation phase, the third stage of the programme. The curve then flattens at just over two pounds per week before dipping below the psychological barrier of two pounds with odd periods of stagnation for women with premenstrual syndrome or if there is any bingeing.

On this subject, you need to know that the body puts up little resistance to the loss of the first few pounds. It has a greater reaction when the plundering of its reserves becomes more threatening. In theory, this would be just the moment to step up your diet. But in practice, the very opposite often occurs. The strongest willpower sometimes weakens in the face of long-suppressed temptations, and invitations to eat out that were once declined are now accepted.

But the real threat comes from elsewhere. The loss of the first 20 pounds brings general visible improvement, shape and suppleness return, breathlessness disappears, compliments come by the dozen, and you have the satisfaction of getting back into clothes that did not fit before. Add to all this the classic excuse of 'just this once', and your wonderful strong determination from the early days suddenly makes way for bingeing followed by a return to drastic dieting, creating a chaotic, yo-yoing situation that soon becomes dangerous.

It is in such circumstances that the overweight person, victorious up until now, risks resting on their laurels, stagnating and ending up abandoning their goal. You have to realize that in the middle of the race, crossing the dangerous territory of weariness and self-satisfaction that are part of any prolonged diet, half of all dieters fall into this trap and let everything slip away.

In this event, there are three ways to react:

- You can abandon the diet, sink into complacency and succumb to compulsive behaviour patterns but with a deep sense of failure that means you quickly put the pounds back on, often going far beyond what you started out with.

- Or you can get back on track after finding your second wind, going back to the Attack diet and sticking with it until your set goal is attained.

- Or you can admit that you feel incapable of going any further, but that you are ready to do whatever it takes to preserve what you have achieved so far. To do this, stop this weight-loss phase of the Dukan Diet and go directly to the Consolidation phase, which has a much more varied choice of food and it is easy to work out how long it lasts (five days for every pound you have lost). Then go to the Stabilization phase, where you are allowed a completely free choice of food, with just one day per week of the pure protein diet.

How Long Should the Diet Last?

The Cruise diet is the most strategic and key time in the slimming period, the one which will take you to your goal, your True Weight. It is what comes into play after the opening salvo of the Attack phase and leads directly to the desired weight determined from the start.

If we look at a case of real obesity with over 40 pounds to lose, if there were no other particular difficulties involved we might hope to shed that weight over 20 weeks of the alternating diet, i.e. in a little under five months.

When the problem is more difficult:

- Either for psychological reasons, little self-discipline or weak motivation.
- Or for physiological reasons, such as a tendency to obesity in the family.
- Or due to personal experience, a history of having dieted many times with bad diets, or diets not followed properly or simply abandoned mid-way.
- Or, finally, for women going through dangerous times as far as their hormones are concerned, during pre-puberty when periods are chaotic, pregnancy and above all during premenopause and menopause and especially if taking hormone replacement therapy that is not well managed.

In all these cases, weight loss will be slowed down and will require specific adjustments. Even so, even in difficult cases, the spirit of the Attack phase is so strong, and the pace of the first two or three weeks so intense, that most resistance and inhibitions are overcome, resulting generally in a loss of eight to ten pounds. This is the point where old demons can reappear to slow things down.

- The patient predisposed to being excessively overweight will fall, in less than a month, under the threshold of losing two pounds a week and reach an acceptable pace of six to seven pounds a month for two to three months. This, added to the initial loss, brings us to about 30 pounds. At this stage, the loss per month will be further reduced, to around four or perhaps three pounds a month. The question asked is simple: is this all worth it? More often than not the answer is no. Except in the case of formal medical advice concerning the threat of diabetes or severe and inoperable arthritis, or an imperative personal reason, it is preferable not to continue and undermine the results obtained, but rather to consolidate and stabilize. We can wait for better days, for a return to a state where the body is calm and can attain the goal set at the very beginning. The results are 35 pounds lost during four months following the alternating protein diet.

- If you are not very motivated or lack willpower, you are in a worse position. You will also lose the first eight to ten pounds, but the temptation to give up will rear its head straightaway. In the best-case scenario, if you can count on those around you and on your doctor helping you, you can expect to lose another ten pounds in five weeks and then quickly go on to the Consolidation phase and even more quickly to the Stabilization phase, where you will have to agree to eat proteins only for just one day a week, for the rest of your life. You have to accept this now, before you even start this programme. Overall result: 22 pounds in two and a half months using the alternating protein diet.

- For those who are immune to dieting because they followed poor diets badly in the past, here is the best solution. The Attack diet acts like a bulldozer, pushing aside all resistance. You, too, will lose 12 pounds during the first three weeks, but, if you follow the instructions precisely for the programme, you will also continue to lose weight without interruption until you actually lose almost 45 pounds in six months using the alternating protein diet. Not very different to the easy case, because your immunity to dieting from your previous diets only affects the proteins with vegetables phases, not the pure protein periods. And you can always start the Dukan Diet again later without any risk of growing weary.

- Women approaching the menopause who go though the premenopause then the actual menopause and face that time in their life when they are most at risk of putting on weight, and especially so if they already have some extra pounds: While going through this long tunnel, which may last ten years or so, from the age of 42 to 52, women have excessive then dissociated hormonal surges, which sometimes suddenly fade away under an avalanche of hot flushes. However, as paradoxical as it may seem, among these women who have a hard time with all this psychological torment, the most determined and dogged fighters are to be found, and you can rely on them to continue right to the end of their diet come what may. For these women, even losing the first few pounds in the Attack phase is a major undertaking. That is why it is vital for them to get their hormone balance under control before starting this programme. This is a matter for the gynaecologist, or family doctor.

Keep in mind that weight gained during the menopause is not irreversible, though it is a difficult period to go through. You will, if armed and ready, get past this difficult stage in six months to a year. If you are taking hormone replacement therapy, and it is well managed – by, for example, starting off with light doses and progressively increasing to whatever best suits you – this is the best way to effectively lose weight. In short, without supervised hormone therapy it can take up to a year to lose around 45 pounds, which may seem a long time but there are many women who manage it. With specialist, well-supervised help, choosing natural hormones and, if necessary anti-aldosterone, which facilitates the elimination of oedema, these 45 pounds can be lost in six to seven months using the alternating protein diet.

Cruise Diet Summary

Keep eating all the Attack diet foods and add the following vegetables, raw or cooked, without restricting quantities, combinations or time of day: tomatoes, cucumbers, radishes, spinach, asparagus, leeks, French beans, cabbage, mushrooms, celery, fennel, all salad greens including chicory, Swiss chard, aubergines, courgettes, peppers. You can even include carrots and beetroot provided you do not eat them at every meal.

Throughout this Cruise phase, you will alternate periods of proteins with vegetables with periods without any vegetables until you reach your desired weight.

PLEASE TAKE NOTE!

If by following my programme, you reach this point on your road map you will have achieved your True Weight – well done. You should realize that as far as the history of your weight is concerned, you are at a point of no return.

Going by my statistics, it is my duty to tell you that:

- Fifty per cent of readers stop here; they consider themselves cured. They forget that there are still two other phases to finish, which alone will ensure that their new weight is maintained over the long term, over a very long time. All those who are impatient will, without exception, put the weight back on or get caught up in chaotic eating that can only end in failure. So you have been warned.

- The other 50 per cent of my readers do not stop here and they follow me into the Consolidation phase. 85 per cent of them go right to the end and achieve a consolidated weight. This is better but not good enough.

- Only those who go on into the fourth and final permanent Stabilization phase, and follow it, achieve the single goal that counts: 'being cured of being overweight'.

- I hope with all my heart, dear reader, that you will not stop here and that you will continue to the very end of our joint undertaking. Otherwise I will have done what has been done for the past 60 years or more; I will have brought you with me into the desert and abandoned you just before you reach the oasis.

The Diet that Consolidates the Weight Lost: a Crucial Transition Phase

You have now arrived at your True Weight, or at the weight you considered acceptable and set as your goal at the start, or at a weight you want to settle for as acceptable or a half-victory, because you know that the effort involved in going further is too much and risks jeopardizing what you have achieved so far.

The time of rigorous constraints is over and you are at last on flat terrain. You and your body have made a prolonged effort and you have been rewarded. But to rest on your laurels now is very dangerous. You have reached a weight that suits you, but this weight that you have achieved does not really quite belong to you yet. You are like a traveller whose train has just pulled into the station to briefly stop in a town. It feels like home to you even though you know nothing about this place and have never lived there. It could all go either way; the train might leave at any time with you aboard, but if you decide to stay, you still have to unload your bags, find somewhere to stay, a job and friends. It is the same situation with the weight you have just lost. Your new weight will truly be yours if you take the time to control it and if you put in the minimum effort required to preserve it.

Get rid of the illusion that you have at last finally taken care of your weight problem and can now go back to your old ways. That would be catastrophic because the same causes lead to the same effects, and in no time at all you will be back to your old weight. I do not mean that you have to continue forever with the aggressive diet that you have just followed. Who would agree to that?

Anyway, the extra pounds that made you follow this diet in the first place, especially if a substantial, or worse, a recurring problem, were certainly no accident. Whether in your genes or an acquired habit, there is something written inside you a bit like the information on a hard disk that will not disappear. So now you have to find a way forward that restricts you as little as possible and incorporate it into your routine so that you do not put any weight back on.

There is a way of doing this and it will be the theme of the fourth phase of the programme, the ultimate Stabilization diet. But you are not there yet because your body is still adapting to the constraints of dieting over the past few months. You are still predisposed to gain weight and this tendency is now actually heightened by your body's defence impulse as it thinks that it has been robbed of its reserves.

What you need to do is to make peace with your body, which is just waiting for the opportunity to replenish those reserves. This is the objective of this next phase, where you consolidate the weight lost and which, when completed, will open the door to every dieter's dream: permanent stabilization at little cost and the one day a week answer that will be the theme of the final stage of the Dukan Diet.

But to be completely ready to start this Consolidation stage, you have to understand why you are still too vulnerable, and your body too exasperated and too prone to weight rebound, for you to move straight to the Stabilization phase. After this brief and vital theoretical explanation we will look in detail at how you follow this Consolidation phase in practice, the new foods it involves and how long it lasts.

The Weight Rebound Reaction

When a body has lost a good number of pounds through effective dieting, several reactions conspire to put the weight back on. How do we explain such reactions? To understand them, you need to know what the build-up of fat reserves means for a normal body. Building up fat reserves when your food intake is more than enough to cover your energy output is an easy way of storing surplus calories, useless for the time being, but which the body wants to have available in case of any future food shortage.

Fat was the simple solution nature came up with to conserve and store energy; it is the most concentrated form known in the animal kingdom (one gram of fat = nine calories). Nowadays, when food is completely and easily accessible, we may well ask ourselves what use this is to us.

But, again, you have to remember that our biological system was not designed for the modern world; it came into being at a time when access to food was hazardous, unpredictable and always required struggle and hard work. Being fat, which we today find embarrassing, was a precious survival tool for the first humans. The human body, whose biological programming has remained unchanged, still bestows the same importance on what it considers as its vital reserves, and does not like to see them being plundered.

A body that is losing weight risks being left with no supplies if there is the slightest interruption in its food supply. That is why it reacts – because it feels threatened biologically. All its reactions have one sole objective: to recover all the fat it has lost as soon as possible. Your body has three very effective ways of doing this:

- The first is to trigger hunger pangs and sharpen your appetite so as to change your eating habits; the more frustrating your diet was, the stronger this reaction will be. On the instinctive and biological level, the greatest frustration is caused by protein powder diets, which if followed for a long time to the exclusion of anything else can result in bulimic episodes and other compulsive eating disorders.
- Your body's second strategy is to reduce its energy consumption. If you earn less money, you tend to spend less. Biological organisms react in a similar way. This is why many patients complain about feeling cold during weight-loss diets; your body is using less energy to keep you warm. The same goes for tiredness: when we feel tired we avoid any unnecessary effort, excessive activity becomes difficult and everything slows down. Memory and intellectual effort, which require a lot of

energy, also feel the effects. The need for sleep and rest, which save energy, also increases. Hair and nails grow less rapidly. In short, in order to adapt to a long period of losing weight, the body goes into a kind of hibernation.

• Finally, the body's third reaction is the most efficient and the most dangerous one, whether you are trying to lose weight or are already stabilizing, as it consists in better assimilating the calories from your food and getting the most out of them. An individual who ordinarily gets 100 calories from a slice of bread will end up, at the end of the diet, with 120–130 from the same slice. Each morsel is sifted through and everything possible is absorbed. This increase in calorie extraction takes place in the small intestine, the interface between the food (exterior) and the blood (interior).

Increase in appetite, reduction in energy used and maximum extraction of calories consumed all combine to transform the overweight body that has just slimmed down into a calorie sponge. This is usually the moment when you are so happy with your results that you assume you can lower your guard and return to your old habits. This is the most frequent and natural cause for those pounds quickly piling back on again.

So, after you have carefully followed a diet and attained your desired weight this is the time to be most careful. It is called the rebound; like a ball that has just touched the ground, weight has a tendency to bounce back.

How long does the rebound period last?

There is still no natural or therapeutic method today to counter rebound. The best way to protect yourself against it is to know how long it will last, so that during this time you can fight it with the correct eating strategy. Over time I have patiently observed rebound effects among a great many of my patients and have concluded that the high-risk period for regaining weight lasts about five days for every pound lost, 30 days or a month for six to seven pounds, and 100 days for a loss of 18–20 pounds. I attach great importance to this rule, because, here again, it is the lack of precise information that puts you at greatest risk when you have lost weight and finished dieting. Understanding the dangers and how long they last really helps you both to get through the transition period and to more easily accept the additional but crucial effort you will need to make to neutralize the rebound.

The simple passage of time, if you do not relax excessively, allows your system, which is on alert to conserve weight, to settle down and relax. At the end of the tunnel a calm sea and my Stabilization diet await, with its three simple, concrete and painless measures, including the famous protein Thursdays.

Meanwhile, you have to follow a new, more open, diet, not a weight-loss diet because that phase is over; but it is not yet a diet free from all constraints. It does offer freedom, but within limits, its aim being to control your body's excessive reactions and prevent any weight rebound.

How Do I Choose My Correct Stabilization Weight?

It is hard to get into stabilization – even if you are set on doing everything you can to never put back on the weight you have fought so hard to lose – without having a precise weight target and without having defined a future weight objective that is both satisfying and realistic. It is my duty to give you my advice, because I have witnessed too many failures, due in the most part to an unrealistic choice of stabilization weight.

There are a large number of abstract formulas used to come up with your ideal weight according to your height, age, gender and bone structure. All these formulas are theoretically applicable, but I am wary of them, because they are about statistical individuals who in reality do not exist. They do not take into account the particular case of the obese person, who is predisposed to put on weight.

So, in place of a theoretical ideal weight, I tend to use the more realistic notion of the weight that you can stabilize at, because not all weights can be stabilized by any given person. It is not the same thing. The best way to calculate a good stabilization weight is to ask the dieter what weight they can most easily achieve and at which they feel good. There are two reasons for this.

First of all, you have no doubt noticed that it is easier to lose pounds at certain weight levels than at others, and there are extreme areas where whatever diet you follow, your weight is mysteriously blocked. This is when the notion of 'plateau' appears, a plateau that it is difficult to get off. Trying to stabilize your weight in this last area is doomed to fail, because the effort required is disproportionate to the result obtained. And in the unlikely case that you could reach such a weight level, wanting to maintain yourself there would require so much effort it would be unbearable in the long run.

Furthermore, for those who had an awful lot of extra pounds, I place far greater emphasis on wellbeing than on the symbolic value of an abstract and supposedly 'normal' number. If you are predisposed to being overweight you are not just the average person. There is nothing wrong with this, but it means you should not be set a goal that does not suit who you are. What you need is to be able to live normally, happy with a weight that makes you feel good and comfortable with yourself. Keeping this will be a remarkable feat in itself. Finally, you have to bear in mind the maximum and minimum weights you have reached in all your fluctuations, because no matter how long it lasted, it is the maximum weight you reached that your body will have forever recorded in its memory.

Let's take a concrete example. Imagine a woman about five feet six inches tall who has, on just one day of her life, weighed over $15\frac{1}{2}$ stone. It is an absolute impossibility that such a woman could ever hope to stabilize at around eight stone as some theoretical tables would suggest. Her body's biological memory retains the information regarding the maximum weight and this can never be erased. To recommend that she reach and stabilize at 11 stone is more sensible, at least on paper, but only if she already feels comfortable at that weight.

Finally, there is another common double mistake that must be sorted out right away. Many dieters, those who are very overweight as well as those who are not quite so overweight, think that it will be easier to stabilize at a certain weight if they lose a little more so that they have a few pounds as a safety margin to give them some leeway. Wanting, for example, to go down to nine and a half stone in order to stabilize at 11 stone is not just an error, it is a huge mistake, because the amount of willpower wasted getting your weight right down will be sorely missed when you need it later in order to stabilize. Above all, the more you force your weight down, the more your system will be prone to rebound upward.

In conclusion, you must choose a weight that is achievable and at which 'you can stabilize', high enough to be attainable without getting lost on the way, and low enough to provide gratification and the wellbeing you need to stick to it.

I have called this weight the True Weight. It is not the same thing as the BMI, the Body Mass Index (see page 234), which is useful for pinpointing high-risk groups but less so for determining an individual's weight and setting strategic goals.

How do we work out the True Weight?
By definition this weight is personal; to be relevant and workable, it has to take the person's gender and age into account so as to distinguish between a woman's morphotype and that of a man, and above all between

the differences in expectations of being slim that the two sexes have. The same goes for age: we know that with each decade a woman's stable weight has to be increased by 1.8 pounds and a man's by 2.6 pounds. What is more, how can we fail to differentiate between our needs and especially the likelihood of achieving a certain weight when we are 20 or 50 years old?

But when working out this True Weight, family history also has to be considered. Here again, there is no point asking a woman whose family has a history of obesity to aim for the same stable weight as a woman whose family are by nature slim. Furthermore, it is absolutely essential to include the history of the individual's weight problems, the crucial moment when it started to get out of control: was it childhood, adolescence, the first contraceptive pill, pregnancies, the premenopause, major stress, medical treatment, depression? Each case is different from the next and has to be included in what is suggested. It is also equally necessary to take into account what I call the 'weight range', the difference between the least a person has ever weighed after the age of 20 and the most they have weighed apart from during pregnancy. This range tells us what is recorded in the body's biological memory and remains there forever. Also just how many unsuccessful diets have been followed and which ones, as there are some diets from which the body never quite recovers, diets that go against nature and trigger 'body anxieties'. The best known of these are packet or powder substitutes, which are the very opposite of what it is natural for humans to eat. Man is not programmed to feed on powders. He can manage it for a short time but, especially if he loses weight by eating these powders, he may develop a sort of adverse reaction, which unfortunately makes him resistant to other natural methods. Fasting, which amounts to swallowing nothing other than water, is a disaster for our muscle mass as the body has to use it to get the vital proteins it needs for its survival. But fasting is infinitely more natural than eating powders, as it can happen that a predator catches no prey and is forced to fast for a few days.

You can see that there are many different parameters used to calculate the True Weight and that it is crucial to establish what it is in order to work out a road map. It is too complex to be calculated just by using pen and paper. I recommend that you go to my website www.dukandiet.co.uk where you will find a free questionnaire with eleven questions. Answer them and you will have your True Weight straightaway. Then you will know exactly what the bull's-eye is for your target; you can measure the distance, I will give you the bow and arrow and you will stand a much better chance of scoring a hit.

The Transition Diet Day by Day

You have just ended your final day of the alternating protein diet and for the first time on your scales you have seen your True Weight, the weight that I hope you have managed to achieve. If this is not the case, then the weight that you set yourself when you started your diet. Like many others before you, carried away by your success, you feel tempted to continue to try and lose a little more to have a safety margin. Please do not think of doing this. The dice have been thrown, you wanted this weight, you have it and now you have to summon all your strength to try and keep it. I am not just saying this: *one in every two failures occurs in the three months after the desired weight has been attained.*

How Long Should the Diet Last?

The length of this transition diet is based on how much weight you have lost, by calculating five days on this new diet for every pound lost. If you have just lost 40 pounds you have to follow it for 40 times five days, or 200 days (i.e. six months and 20 days); 20 pounds equal 100 days. Everyone can easily calculate the exact amount of time they need until the definitive Stabilization diet begins.

Am I going to give you the Stabilization diet at this point? No, you now realize that you are too vulnerable, you are like a deep-sea diver coming up from the depths who has to do it in stages for safety's sake. This is the role of the diet that I am now going to introduce.

During this Consolidation period, you will follow as faithfully as possible the following diet when you can eat as much as you want from the following foods:

Proteins and vegetables

Up to this point, during your entire Cruise diet, you alternated between proteins and proteins + vegetables, so you are now very familiar with these two food categories. From now on, you do not have to alternate. You can eat all proteins and vegetables together and still have as much as you want.

Proteins and vegetables constitute a complete, stable foundation on which, from now on, you will build the Consolidation phase that we are going to talk about here, as well as the final and permanent Stabilization phase that will follow it. You can see why these two major food categories are so important, because for the rest of your life you can eat them without there being any limit on quantity, time of day or combination.

You probably know all the foods by now, but I will briefly review them so as to avoid any misunderstanding. For more details, you will find the complete list in the sections on the Attack diet and the alternating protein diet. They are:

- lean meats – the least fatty cuts of beef and veal
- offal
- fish and seafood
- poultry (except duck and goose) and always without the skin
- low-fat ham, sliced low-fat chicken and turkey
- plant proteins
- eggs
- non-fat dairy products

- raw and cooked vegetables
- one and a half litres of water

As well as the above base of proteins and vegetables now familiar to you, your Consolidation introduces new foods that will improve your daily eating. They can be added in the following proportions and quantities.

One serving of fruit per day

The opportunity now arises to talk about a food that most of you believe belongs to the 'as much as you want' category, because it is so naturally healthy.

This is partly true: fruit *is* a natural product and free from toxicity. It is also one of the best-known sources of vitamin C and carotene.

But these advantages have been mythologized by two recent Western preoccupations: our longing to return to what is natural and our belief in the magical virtues of vitamins. However, just being natural does not automatically mean beneficial and vitamins are not quite the magical solution that many seem to think they are.

In fact, fruit is the only natural food that contains what diabetes specialists call rapid assimilation sugars. All other sources of sugar are man-made.

Honey is, in fact, a surreptitious food, an animal secretion, a sort of growth milk intended only for immature bees, but which we enjoy for its taste. Refined sugar, white sugar, does not exist as such in nature as it is an artificial food made from sugar cane or sugar beet.

Fruit in its natural state was a precious food that for a long time mostly decorated the table, a colourful and satisfying reward for man. It is only through intensive farming and selection that we nowadays have the impression that fruit is easy to come by. As it is, most fruit with a high sugar content, such as oranges, bananas and mangos, comes to us from faraway tropical regions and was only recently introduced into our regular diet, thanks to progress in transportation. This explains certain serious allergies, occasionally deadly, to some exotic fruits, such as peanuts or kiwi fruit.

In fact, fruit is not the prototype of healthy and natural food. Consumed in large quantities it can be dangerous, especially for diabetics and overweight people who tend to eat fruit outside mealtimes.

Rationed to one fruit per day, you are now allowed to eat all fruit, except bananas, grapes, cherries, dried fruits and nuts (walnuts, peanuts, almonds, pistachios and cashews).

As for servings, this is usually a single unit for fruit the size of an apple, pear, orange, grapefruit, peach or nectarine. For smaller fruits, or larger ones, use a normal serving: a bowl of strawberries or raspberries, a slice of cantaloupe or honeydew melon, a decent slice of watermelon, two kiwis, two nice apricots, one small mango or half a large one. You can eat all these fruits but remember one serving per day and not per meal.

However, when you can choose according to your own preferences, bear in mind that the best fruits for your stabilization are the following, in descending order: priority is given to the apple, because its high pectin content helps keep your figure trim; strawberries and raspberries are low in calories and look colourful and festive; if you stick to the serving size, melon and watermelon for their high water and low calorie content; grapefruit then, finally, kiwi, peach, pear, nectarine and mango.

Two slices of wholemeal bread per day

If you are prone to put on weight, get into the habit of avoiding white bread. Because of the way it is produced it is not a natural food; the flour used comes from wheat stripped of its husk, the bran. This makes obtaining industrial flours easier, but the bread produced from them is too refined; it is not a natural product and enters into the bloodstream too quickly and in too great a quantity.

Wholemeal bread, which also tastes good, has a natural proportion of bran, which is a major ally. Its plant-like structure and fibrous framework are solid enough to resist your digestion's fire power. Because of this it speeds digestion and creates a protective screen in the colon between the intestinal lining and dangerous waste products that stagnate and build up there.

Take care! Don't confuse the wheat bran in bread with oat bran. Wheat bran in wholemeal bread is an insoluble fibre, whereas oat bran is highly soluble. This means it can swell in the stomach and distend it until it feels satisfied, and, what is more, it can trap nutrients and their calories in the intestines so that they pass out together in the stools.

For this phase of the diet, you are still under strict surveillance as your body is waiting to extract calories from everything. But once you reach the permanent Stabilization stage, you will be able to eat bread normally, as long as it is wholegrain or, even better, bread enriched with bran. From now on, if you enjoy bread at breakfast, you may lightly spread your two slices of wholemeal bread with some fat-reduced butter. But you may also decide to eat these two slices of bread at some other time of the day, for a cold meat or ham sandwich at lunchtime, or in the evening with some cheese, which is the next food to be added to your list.

One serving of cheese per day
What cheese are you allowed to eat and how much?

You may eat all hard rind cheeses such as Cheddar, Swiss cheese, Gouda and other cheeses from Holland, Tomme de Savoie (a hard French cheese from the Alps), Mimolette, Emmental, etc. Avoid fermented cheese for now, such as blue cheese, Brie, Camembert or goat's cheese. As for how much, you should eat a 40g (1½oz) serving. I am not usually in favour of weighing food, but since this phase of the diet will not last too long, this is a good standard serving that satisfies most appetites. Choose whichever meal suits you best, but remember only one serving per day.

What about fat-reduced or diet cheeses? Many are of poor quality so if you cannot find a good one, I would advise against eating food that has lost most of its flavour.

As for the great and refined cheeses, true works of art for the palate for which the French are justly famous, rest assured they are not totally forbidden. Just be patient, because shortly you will be pleasantly surprised by the special celebration meals.

Two servings of 'starchy' foods per week

Up until now you have been allowed to eat the reintroduced foods every day. With starchy foods and then celebration meals, it will be on a weekly basis. Moreover, for these two important new elements you will have to approach this Consolidation phase **in two parts**. After calculating how long it will last, based on five days for every pound lost, divide this phase into two equal parts: the first and the second. In the first you are allowed one portion of starchy foods per week and in the second both together, which avoids the risk of you starting to eat sugar-rich foods too suddenly.

Let's get back to our starchy foods. For a long time this term used to refer only to potatoes, but now we also use it to include foods made from flour, such as breads and pasta, as well as cereals such as rice and corn. In our Consolidation phase, where prudence is the rule, all starches are not of equal value, and I list them for you here in descending order of interest.

- Pasta is the starch best adapted for our particular use; at least pasta made with hard wheat whose vegetable texture is very resistant, much more so than other varieties. This resistance to being broken down slows digestion and the absorption of sugar. Moreover, everyone likes pasta and it is rarely associated with dieting, so it is a source of comfort for dieters who have been working so hard to lose weight. Finally, and most importantly, pasta has a filling and satisfying consistency. Its only drawback is that it is often cooked with butter, oil or cream as well as cheese, which then doubles the calorie intake. So eat pasta, and take a proper 225g (8oz) serving but avoid oil and opt instead for a nice sauce of fresh tomatoes, onions and spices. If you are in a hurry, use tomato paste or canned tomatoes. As for cheese, avoid Swiss cheese, which is too fatty and you end up using more because of its bland taste. Instead, try a light sprinkling of Parmesan, which is both far less rich and stronger tasting – the Italians know a thing or two!

- Couscous, bulgur wheat, polenta and Ebly durum wheat: Also made from hard wheat and with the same beneficial properties as pasta, these foods are generally less well known and used because they come from foreign cultures.

Couscous is often thought of as being complicated to make and best enjoyed in restaurants. But why deprive yourself unnecessarily of a food that is very good for stabilization? To prepare it quickly, put the couscous in a non-metallic bowl and add some hot bouillon made with a cube of your choice until it is covered, with 5mm (¼in) of liquid to spare. Let the grain absorb the liquid and swell up for five minutes. Put the couscous in a microwave for one minute, then take it out and mix it with a fork to break up any lumps. Put it back in the microwave for another minute and then it is ready. Do not add any oil or butter, and do not order couscous in a restaurant as it is usually drowned in butter.

You may eat the same quantity – 225g (8oz) portions – of Italian polenta, Lebanese bulgur wheat and other durum wheat such as Ebly prepared in the same way.

- Lentils, with one of the slowest sugars around, are another good choice. Unfortunately, they do take time to prepare, are not universally popular and, what is worse, they have a reputation for causing flatulence. But for those who like them and digest them well, they are an excellent stabilization food and very satisfying. You are allowed a 225g (8oz) serving. Once again, no oil, but do serve with tomatoes, onions and spices – a bay leaf works well.

  Other beans also deserve to be mentioned and you are allowed the same quantity prepared without oil. Haricot beans, butter beans, dried peas, chick peas, split peas and dried beans of all colours belong to the same family. Some people find them difficult but they all provide excellent nutrition.

- Rice and potatoes are also allowed, but, as you can see, appear at the bottom of our list and so can only be eaten occasionally. Priority should be given to the foods listed above. However, unless you are in a Chinese or Japanese restaurant, it is better to eat brown rice, without butter or oil, as it is assimilated more slowly because of its fibre. Or choose the tastier varieties such as basmati and wild rice. Each serving must not exceed 175g (6oz) of white rice or 225g (8oz) of brown rice, cooked and weighed.

As for potatoes, prepare them baked in their skin in aluminium foil, or boiled, and always without any butter or sauce. Chips or, even worse, crisps feature among the few foods that I advise you to forget about totally, not only because they are full of fat and calories, but because they are dangerous if you want to prevent cardiovascular illness and cancer.

New meats you can add to your diet
Up until now you were allowed the lean parts of beef and veal. From now on you can add lamb and roast pork as well as ham, in any quantity, once or twice a week.

- Leg of lamb is the leanest part of the animal. But avoid eating the outer slices of the roast; there are two good reasons for this. Firstly, the fat surrounding the leg of lamb does not come away easily so there is always some remaining which makes the first slice high in fat and calories. Secondly, large roasts are usually cooked with a very high surface temperature to ensure that they are properly cooked inside. But this often chars the outside layer, making it carcinogenic. If you like your meat well done, take the second slice.

- Roast pork is likewise allowed because roast joints

are usually the least fatty part of the animal, but avoid cuts from along the spine because they are twice as fatty.

- Cooked ham may now be eaten. You are no longer limited solely to rind-less extra-lean ham. You may eat all kinds of ham, but be careful to remove all fat. However, avoid cured hams such as Parma ham, which are not allowed yet.

So these are the food categories that are the platform for your transition diet. Remember that this is not at all a permanent diet or a weight-loss diet. This is a healthy, balanced diet whose only role is to help you get through a tumultuous period when your body, worried about losing its reserves, is doing all it can to restore them.

Five days for every pound lost is about the time you need to reassure your body and for it to come to terms with the new weight you are trying to impose on it. Once you get beyond this transition period, you will be free again to eat how you want for six days out of seven. This prospect should give you the encouragement and patience you need; you know where you are heading and how long it will take.

But that is not all. To conclude this transition diet, I have two more important things to tell you, some good news and some necessary information. I will start with the good news.

Two Celebration Meals a Week

As I explained for starchy foods, during the first half of the Consolidation phase you are allowed one celebration meal per week, increasing to two during the second half. So that you do not make a mistake I will give you a simple example: you have just lost 20 pounds, so your Consolidation phase will have to last 100 days. Divide these 100 days into two equal 50-day sections. The first 50 days, you are allowed one portion of starchy foods and one celebration meal per week. For the remaining 50 days, two portions of starchy foods and two celebration meals. I really want to emphasize the word 'meal' here because even when I write it out on a prescription some patients read this and seem to think that it means 'all day long'.

What is a celebration meal? A celebration meal can be any one of your three meals in the day, but my advice is to choose dinner so that you can enjoy it and avoid any work stress that may overshadow breakfast and lunch.

Celebration means party-time! At each of these two meals you can eat whatever kind of food you want and especially whatever you have most missed during the weight-loss period. There are nevertheless two important conditions: never have second helpings of the same dish, and never eat two celebration meals in a row. Everything is allowed, but one of each: one starter, one main dish, one dessert, and one glass of wine; all in a reasonable quantity but only once.

Take care to space out these meals and give your body

time to recover. If you have a celebration meal for lunch on Tuesday, then do not have one for dinner on the same day. Leave at least one meal in between. You might also want to keep them for evenings and weekends when you are eating out.

For those of you who miss steak and kidney pie, curry, paella or any other dish now is your chance. For those of you who have been waiting so long to finish your meal with a real dessert, such as a piece of chocolate cake, or ice cream, well now you can. For those of you who like good wine or champagne, you can now enjoy them too.

Now, without a second thought you can at long last accept those dinner invitations you have had to refuse, but only once, then twice, a week.

Many of you who have got this far, to the Stabilization phase, will have become so used to eating in a new way that you hesitate to let go and enjoy a celebration meal.

You should understand that these meals too have been carefully planned and are part of a whole, so although they might seem excessive the end result is balance and equilibrium. Moreover, these celebration meals are not simply suggestions, they are instructions you must follow to the letter. The Dukan Diet is a comprehensive programme and you cannot pick and choose from its different component parts without reducing its effectiveness. Maybe you do not fully understand why the freedom of these two meals is so important. Now, then, is the time to talk to you about pleasure, the other aspect of eating.

Nourishing yourself is not just about taking in enough calories to survive; it is also, and even more importantly, about enjoying eating as part of that process. It is now time to reintroduce this biological pleasure, this vital reward which was taken away from you during your weight-loss period.

Since we are talking about what tastes good, I will use this opportunity to give you an important piece of advice, essential for any permanent stabilization. So do not take it lightly.

When you eat, and particularly if what you are eating is savoury and rich, THINK ABOUT WHAT YOU ARE EATING, concentrate on what is in your mouth and on each and every sensation this food is giving you. Numerous studies carried out by nutritionists prove the major role that taste sensations play in making us feel full. All taste sensations, from the tongue's mucous secretions and each movement of chewing and swallowing, are analyzed by the hypothalamus, the centre in the brain responsible for hunger and satisfaction. The accumulation of these sensations raises a sensory gauge that, at a certain point, triggers the feeling of being full and satisfied.

SO EAT SLOWLY and CONCENTRATE ON WHAT IS IN YOUR MOUTH. Avoid eating while watching television or reading, because you reduce the intensity of the sensations going to your brain, which is being distracted by images and words. Nutritionists explain the obesity epidemic in children by the fact that they eat and snack in front of the TV for hours every day and then as grown-ups continue to eat all day long.

Enjoy these two wonderful celebration-meal moments, without any guilt or afterthoughts, and, believe me, they will not cost you a thing.

There are, however, two conditions you must abide by:

- The first is of utmost importance. This freedom is precisely limited in time. For now, it is only one and then a second meal. Not sticking to these limits would lead you off the route we have been taking. Do not play down the danger. If you have chosen Tuesday night, for example, for your celebration meal, you need to understand that Wednesday's breakfast is when the success of your diet is on the line.

  Having opened the door to whatever you want, will you have the courage to close it again, or will you be one of those people unable to resist spreading jam all over their toast?

  These two celebration freedom meals are the frills that brighten up your humdrum daily diet and are there to help you hold on until your body accepts its new weight. They are an integral part of your transition diet which I have devised by including what I could for you. But if you step beyond these limits, you risk compromising everything that you have so patiently worked for.

- The second condition is common sense. The celebration meal is meant to give you a dose of pleasure, but is not an invitation to binge. Anyone who uses this freedom as an excuse to stuff themselves has not understood me and runs the risk of damaging their system. The real goal of these two meals is to give you a certain equilibrium. Eating until you are nauseous or drinking until you are drunk will throw you completely off balance. Even if you go back on the straight and narrow the next day, back to the consolidation platform, the rhythm will have been broken and with it your hope of eventual stabilization.

If you want a simple piece of advice, eat what you want, give yourself generous servings, but never take seconds. If you eat your celebration meal at home or at a friend's home, do as you would in a restaurant, where you cannot ask for a second helping.

One Day of Pure Proteins Per Week: Thursdays

Here you are with all of the ingredients that make up the Dukan Diet's Consolidation phase. You know now what you have to eat and how long this period, easily calculated, will last until your body accepts the new weight imposed on it.

Nevertheless, one key ingredient, vital for the security of this Stabilization phase, is missing. This diet, with the added variety of two celebration meals a week, cannot on its own guarantee perfect weight control during this highly sensitive period. That is why, at the heart of this Consolidation phase, I have included, by way of security, one full day per week of the pure protein diet, which you have already tried and tested.

On this day, you will revert to eating just protein-rich foods; you have eaten enough of them to be totally familiar with them. I will just remind you of the main categories: lean meats, offal, all fish and seafood, poultry without the skin, extra-lean hams, plant proteins, eggs, non-fat dairy products and two litres of water. As before, you can eat as much and as often as you want from these protein categories and in any combination and proportions that suit you.

This pure protein day is both the driving force and insurance policy for your Consolidation phase. This will then be the sole constraint you face during the week, but it is also the price you need to pay during the Stabilization phase to keep things under control until the storm is over.

Again, this price is not negotiable. Carry out this day to the letter or do not do it at all, but you are the one who will lose out.

If possible, always make it a set day, Thursday for example. This weekly rhythm is one of the guarantees of its effectiveness. If Thursdays are not possible for you because of your job or social schedule, make it Wednesday or Friday and stick to it.

If for some reason you cannot keep to your pure protein day on the Thursday, do it the previous or the next day and the following week go back to your chosen day. But do not slip into the habit of breaking the rhythm this way.

Do not forget that you are predisposed to putting on

weight. You are not doing this to please me but to fight against your own tendency to put on the pounds easily. You are the one who will benefit from following this rule, so remember that.

If you are on holiday or travelling, keep it up. If you are somewhere where it is hard to find protein foods or they are difficult to prepare, you can resort to protein powder if nothing else is available. I will talk more about this later. It is a simple way, on the odd occasion, of making this day as effective as possible.

Oat bran

During the Consolidation phase, you must keep eating two tablespoons of oat bran per day. These two tablespoons are in addition to the two slices of bread and if you have become used to having a galette for breakfast, keep the bread to have in the evening with the cheese.

Exercise

During the Consolidation phase, you can lower the walking time to 25 minutes a day. Obviously, this is the minimum compulsory duration but if you enjoy it and have the time then walk for longer. Walking is one of the most useful human activities, for the number of calories it burns up – as you are likely to keep on doing it in the long term – and also for your wellbeing. As well as being a most natural human activity, it is also the one that results in the greatest secretion of serotonin and endorphins, two transmitter substances behind pleasure and fulfilment and the biological signs of happiness.

If you are dealing with stress or frustration, if you are suffering from depression or nervous exhaustion, if you have been hurt, if you feel abandoned or on your own, go for a walk and take pleasure in what you see, what you come across and who you meet, and I promise you that you will come back feeling better than when you set out.

Do Not Overlook this Phase

We have now finished describing the Consolidation phase. I have kept until the end four pieces of advice to warn you of the dangers of neglecting this crucial stage in the Dukan Diet.

A crucial stage

During this third phase of the Dukan Diet, you will not have the encouragement and excitement of watching your weight go down on the scales. You might therefore start wondering why you have to follow this intermediate diet where you are not yet really free but not losing weight either. You could be tempted to relax your self-control or simply go beyond recommended limits.

Do not do this. If you neglect this consolidation stage then there is one thing you can be absolutely sure of: all those pounds you lost with such effort will most definitely return and return quickly. And if you do not put on a few extra too you will be getting off lightly.

Progressive resistance to dieting

Besides the feeling of frustration and defeat produced by putting weight back on, there is another more serious danger with far-reaching consequences for those who follow diets without consolidating them: resistance to dieting altogether.

Anyone who loses and regains weight several times during their life becomes immune to dieting; that is to say that after each defeat it becomes increasingly difficult to lose weight again. The body has a sort of memory of the diets it has been through and finds better ways of resisting new attempts to lose weight. So each defeat opens the door to another one. If you have already tried other diets in vain, do not expect to lose weight as quickly as someone who is dieting for the first time, even if, as I have already explained, the first two phases of my programme make up the diet duo that encounters the least resistance and best attacks any immunity to previous dieting.

Memory of weight extremes

Moreover, every time you put on weight and reach a new record number on your scales, the way your physiology adjusts means that somewhere in your brain, a sort of nostalgic memory of this maximum weight is recorded, which your body will then always try to reach again.

Losing weight is the same as feeding yourself with fat and cholesterol

Finally and probably the most serious of these consequences is that with each weight loss, your body suffers an attack which many of you may not be aware of. Each attempt to lose weight makes you consume your fat reserves and when you lose 20 or 40 pounds, it is almost as if you had eaten that amount of fat or butter.

Throughout this weight-loss period, a large quantity of cholesterol circulates in your blood, along with triglycerides. Each time your heart contracts, this blood, rich in toxic fats, inundates the arteries and coats their inner walls.

Losing weight might be very useful for both your psychological and physical wellbeing and the risks posed by these circulating fats are largely compensated for by such benefits. But be careful not to try and lose weight too often, especially if using rather feeble diets that you know in your heart will never ever be stabilized. People who try to lose weight without success once or twice a year are constantly exposing themselves to high levels of cholesterol. This is not meant to frighten you, but to warn you about a very real danger, one that both doctors and their patients are little aware of.

You have succeeded in losing weight, and now for all the reasons mentioned you must make the only logical choice, which is to consolidate the new weight you have worked so hard to achieve and then move on, as scheduled, to permanent stabilization.

Consolidation Diet Summary

How long this transition diet lasts is calculated according to how much weight you have lost, based on five days for every pound shed. If you have just lost 40 pounds, you have to follow it for 40 times five days, i.e. 200 days or six months and 20 days; 20 pounds is equivalent to 100 days. You can easily calculate the exact amount of time you need before reaching permanent stabilization.

The whole time you are consolidating your weight, you will follow this diet as closely as possible and you are allowed the following foods:

- the protein foods from the Attack diet
- the vegetables from the Cruise diet
- one serving of fruit per day, except bananas, raisins and cherries
- two slices of wholemeal bread per day
- 40g (1½oz) cheese per day
- two servings of starchy foods per week
- lamb and pork roast (lean cuts)

Then to crown it all:
- two celebration meals per week (you are free to choose, but no bingeing)

But also, absolutely and without question:
- one day of pure proteins (the Attack diet) per week, on the same day every week and without fail
- two tablespoons of oat bran per day
- 25 minutes of walking per day

How to Stabilize Your Weight Once and For All

If you began my programme considerably overweight, let's now take stock. The Attack diet gave you an encouraging and lightning kick-start, the Cruise diet guided you to your target weight and now you have just completed your Consolidation diet based on five days for every pound lost.

At this stage, you have not only got rid of your extra pounds, but you have also made it safely through the period during which your new slimmed body was trying with all its might to recover those lost pounds.

Before, you had achieved your True Weight and now you have also consolidated it. This means that your body is no longer extremely defensive. It has given up this extreme reactivity, wanting to extract every last calorie from everything you eat. Your metabolism is once again calmer. Nevertheless it remains very clever at extracting what it can and putting on weight, as it has gone through all those times when you have gained weight in the past. From now on, since the same causes produce the same effects, the likelihood of regaining weight will remain if you do not incorporate into your lifestyle a certain number of habits specifically designed to deal with this risk.

But, and here is the danger, it is now no longer a question of going through a period of constraint with exact instructions, but simply a matter of returning to a normal lifestyle with the freedom to eat what you want. What is more, the measures that I am asking you to adopt in this permanent stabilization programme will have to become part of your way of life for the rest of your life. So, with that in mind, it makes no sense to impose heavy constraints on you that you could never manage to keep.

Most importantly, you have been guided up until now by a whole system of precise instructions. You took up a challenge that left no room for improvisation. From this moment, instead of sailing along the coastline, you will be out on the open seas, with much more independence than before, but also exposed to a greater risk of storms and, therefore, of shipwreck. So it is important that these new instructions are sufficiently simple, concrete and painless to become part of your way of life.

To do this, and to break the cycle of putting the lost weight back on as soon as the dieting is finished, permanent stabilization offers you, in return for four simple and not-too-frustrating measures, freedom to eat again whatever you want so that you no longer feel excluded at mealtimes.

The first of these measures is simple: all you need do is adopt the basic foods from the Consolidation phase as a safety platform. As much as you want of all the protein foods and vegetables, a piece of fruit, two slices of wholemeal bread, 40g (1½oz) of cheese, two portions of starchy foods and two celebration meals. These foods comprise a healthy, copious and sufficiently varied range to constitute the basis for a human diet. Use this as your point of reference and in particular as your safety back-up where you can return to take shelter if you are under threat or regaining

144

weight. You already know the second measure, protein Thursdays, as it featured in the Consolidation phase. The third is quite simply a contract between you and me where you promise me that you will no longer take any lifts or escalators and that you will walk for 20 minutes a day. And the final measure is simply a treat: you must stick to three tablespoons of oat bran a day for life.

Together, these measures seem to me the least disagreeable things you could be asked to do in return for being able to eat normally six days out of seven. My professional experience leads me to believe that no sensible person who wants to avoid becoming overweight again could refuse such a deal.

In addition, to crown these measures, the Dukan Diet's permanent stabilization is protected by an additional weapon, less visible, but decisive: the power of everything you have learnt about nutrition during the time you spent losing pounds then consolidating your new weight.

As I created the programme and use it every day with my patients, I know that every overweight or obese person who has lost 10, 20, 30, 40 or even 60 pounds by following the four successive diets has acquired knowledge about the value of different foods and how to eat that becomes instinctive and deeply ingrained, and this can help them stay slim and stable. They have gained reflexes that they will never quite lose.

Attacking with the pure protein diet, you will have discovered the power of these **vital foods** when selected in such a way as to exclude the two other food groups.

You now know that, combined, these foods represent an extremely effective weapon in the battle to lose weight that you can call upon throughout your life.

Throughout the alternating protein diet, you learned that adding green vegetables slowed down the pace of weight loss, but that these **indispensable foods** did not prevent your pounds continuing to disappear as long as the vegetables were prepared without any fat, a serious enemy unmasked as soon there are any unfortunate lapses in the diet.

When going through consolidation, you included in successive steps such **necessary foods** as bread, fruit, cheese, some starchy foods and even, with your celebration meals, some **pleasurable** and **superfluous foods** without any pangs of guilt. By doing this, in flesh and spirit, day by day, you have incorporated a hierarchy of values and learnt how to classify foods.

It is this progression from different levels, from the **vital** to the **superfluous**, and the instinctive training you have acquired that make this programme the most educational diet there is, which, combined with our other measures for permanent stabilization, leads the way to a solution that may never have been achieved before: weight that is lost and lost permanently.

Protein Thursdays

Why Thursdays?

At that time in my life when I was still putting together the different pieces of what was to become the programme and method that you are now holding, I sensed the need to add one remaining guideline to this stabilization of the lost weight, a final link of protection and friendship, connecting me in thought and deed to my patient or my reader and which would remind them of the battle we had fought together.

In fact, it was one of my patients who gave me the idea. Happy to have lost lots of weight without having suffered as much as she had expected, she was wary of returning to 'normal life' and did not want to completely give up the Attack diet, which helped her to 'put right lapses' whenever she had any. To negotiate the best she could, she came up with this simple and clever argument: 'if only for one day a week!' The idea worked because a few weeks later I decided to experiment by formally writing it out on my prescriptions: 'One day of the pure proteins diet per week.' I observed that this instruction was successfully followed for a certain period of time, then less regularly, and finally, it was forgotten altogether.

So I decided to lay down which day it should be and arbitrarily chose Thursdays. From then on, as if by magic, everything suddenly changed. My patients followed the rule and stuck to it, simply because it was not up to them to choose the day and because nothing is harder for a person with weight problems than to have to choose themselves exactly when they are to be deprived of food. Prescribing a non-negotiable day highlights the importance of this day, which like a barrier holds in check any mishaps during the rest of the week, and that it is too important for the person following the programme to be left to decide. If Thursdays do not work for you, then choose another day of the week but stick to it.

What is special about protein Thursday and how is it different from other protein days?

During the Attack phase, with which you started your diet, I described the 72 foods that made it up – the foods that we call pure protein foods, which you used on their own for the first few days to enhance results. You kept them but alternated them with added vegetables during the Cruise diet. In consolidation, you kept to them for one day a week to counterbalance the introduction of a great number of everyday foods. All this time, you were supported and protected by a whole system of precise instructions that left little room for initiative or error.

From now on you have no safety net.

You may now eat normally six days out of seven and these protein Thursdays are the sole remaining barrier keeping you from your tendency to put on weight. In other words, you must follow these protein days to the letter, because a single weakness or error will threaten their effectiveness and the solidity of all you have achieved.

The foods you are allowed on these Thursdays do not all have the same protein content. For this day, so crucial for your permanent stabilization, we must select and use by choice the purest forms of protein, which, together, produce the most powerful results, and restrict or avoid any that contain some fat and carbohydrates, which if eaten to excess would wipe out the impact these days have.

Protein Thursdays in practice: foods you can choose from

- Lean meat. You already know that pork and lamb are too rich in fat to be counted as pure proteins. Of those that are allowed, veal scores the best but is often expensive and hard to find. Only use the lean parts, which should be grilled or braised. Roasted veal is allowed if well cooked. Veal chops are fattier and can be eaten on other days of the week.

  Beef varies in fat content according to the cut. Apart from fatty cuts for stewing, ribs and rib eye are without doubt the highest in fat and cannot possibly be included in our lean meat category.

  Steaks and T-bone steaks are probably the leanest cuts of beef. You can even find frozen beefburgers and mince with no more than five per cent fat. You can use all of these without a second thought on Thursdays.

  On the other hand, be careful with other cuts if you are unsure of their fat content. If in doubt, ask your butcher.

  You should also know that for protein Thursdays, beef should be well cooked rather than rare. This does not alter the protein content but it does eliminate some of the fat.

  If you can find rabbit, it is an excellent source of pure protein. But do not add mustard sauce on Thursdays as recommended for the Attack diet, but feel free to add a non-fat fromage frais or quark sauce with spices.

- Fish and seafood. In the standard pure protein diet I allowed you to eat all kinds of fish, from the leanest to the fattiest. Over time I have come to accept oily fish such as salmon, sardines, mackerel and tuna, as they are prized for their immense protective power against heart disease and arteriosclerosis and their fat content is no higher than some cuts of meat. Nevertheless, this high fat content, acceptable for the rest of the Dukan Diet, is not so for protein Thursdays, which are your last protective barrier. If you eat salmon, do not eat more than 225g (8oz) per meal if it is fresh, and 175g (6oz) if it is smoked. White fish is your best ally on Thursdays.

As well as the traditional ways of preparing fish, such as poaching, baking, grilling or in a pan, another simple way is to eat it raw. Grouper, bream, sea bass, cod and monkfish are excellent eaten this way. Marinate in thin slices, like sashimi, or cubed, for a few minutes in lemon juice, with some salt, black pepper and herbes de Provence. They make an unusual, fresh and flavourful starter or main course.

Turbot, red mullet and skate are the fattiest white fish but much less so than the leanest meat so you can eat as much of them as you want.

Crab, shrimps, mussels, oysters and scallops are even leaner than fish. A seafood dish or platter can save you from embarrassment if you have to accept an invitation to eat out on a Thursday. However, if you are a fan of shellfish and you like it in great quantities, avoid very fatty oysters, usually the large ones. Add lemon to them, but do not drink their juice.

- Poultry. With the exception of flat-beaked birds such as duck and goose, and when eaten without skin, poultry is one of the best foundations for a protein diet. However, on protein Thursdays, a few words of caution need to temper this freedom.

  Chicken, our basic poultry food, can be eaten freely, but, as well as the skin, avoid the wings, thighs and parson's nose, which can be saved for the rest of the week.

  Other poultry is allowed without any restrictions. Turkey and guinea fowl are the leanest poultry of all, so eat them freely. Pigeon and quail add a festive touch to your protein Thursdays. These birds can all be prepared differently. Chicken is best served oven roasted or on skewers. On Thursdays, go for the skewered kebab version and make sure you remove it from the dish right away so that it does not soak up too much juice and extra fat. Turkey and guinea fowl can be roasted in the oven, moistened occasionally with lemon water so as to separate the fat.

  On Thursdays, the best way to do pigeon or quail is on skewers.
- Eggs. Egg white is the richest natural source of protein, much purer than any protein powder you can buy. But this is only one part of the egg, and the yolk, intended for the growing chick, contains many complex fats, including cholesterol. Together the whole egg provides a balanced food you can eat on Thursdays.

However, if you are finding it hard to stabilize your weight, or if your week has been particularly indulgent and you want to get the maximum impact from your protein Thursday, eat fewer eggs; or, alternatively, avoid the yolk and eat as many whites as you want.

Another solution is to make omelettes or scrambled eggs with one yolk for two whites, and, if you are really hungry, add some powdered skimmed milk. But remember that all these precautions are wasted if you cook your eggs with butter or oil. Get a good quality non-stick frying pan and put a few drops of water in the bottom before breaking your eggs.

- Plant proteins. Tofu and seitan are low in fat and both can be eaten on protein Thursdays.
- Non-fat dairy products. Non-fat fromage frais, quark, yoghurt and cottage cheese have the advantage of having no fat. But what else is in these products which, statistics show, are becoming increasingly popular every year? There is, of course, milk protein which is used to make protein powder, but we also find in moderate quantities lactose, or milk sugar, which is not welcome here.

Our two Attack and Cruise weight-loss diets proved that the presence of lactose does not lessen the pure protein diet's performance and that non-fat milk products, as your only source of fresh and creamy tastes, can be eaten without limit or at least without exceeding around 675g (1½lb) per day. However, for the once-a-week-only protein Thursdays in the permanent Stabilization diet these products must be selected more carefully to reduce your lactose intake. Compare your non-fat cottage cheese, fromage frais, quark and yoghurts and check that for the same number of calories you are getting more protein and less lactose. On Thursdays, if you like dairy products, then go for as little lactose as possible; you can be less fussy the other six days of the week.

- Water. Here, again, we need to adjust the pure protein diet instructions. A litre and a half of water a day is a good minimum amount to purify a body that is burning up its own fat. On these stabilizing Thursdays, you should up this to at least two litres for the day, as this amount will flood the small intestine and reduce its craving for food. Further diluting the food eaten prolongs and slows down its absorption, and another advantage is that digestion is speeded up.

  Thoroughly flushing out the intestines like this, along with the pure proteins, creates a kind of shock wave, whose aim is not only to stop food being assimilated on Thursdays, but also to keep the effect going for the next two or three days. Leaving us then with only three or four days when the energy extracted from your food will be at its highest rate.

- Salt. Salt is an indispensable food. Our body is bathed in a kind of inner fluid (blood and lymph), whose salt level is close to that of the sea. But salt is an enemy for anyone wanting to keep the pounds off. If too much is absorbed, salt retains water and invades tissues already overloaded with fat.

On the other hand, a weight-loss diet lacking in salt can result in lower blood pressure and can cause tiredness if followed for too long. Because of that, the Dukan Diet dictates only a slight reduction in salt during the first three phases.

But for stabilization Thursdays, instructions are stepped up and salt reduced. Restricting intake for one day is not enough to lower blood pressure but it is sufficient to enable the water you drink to pass through your system and clean it out. Purifying tissues is particularly important for women who, because of hormonal influences, experience significant water retention at certain times in their menstrual cycle.

For the same reasons, you should limit mustard on Thursdays, but you can use vinegar, pepper and all other spices to compensate for any lack of flavour.

Powdered Proteins

Up until now, protein has meant natural foods. But, apart from egg white, no food is pure protein per se, so all our efforts have gone into choosing foods with the best protein content.

The food industry has for some time now offered powdered proteins, close to total purity. In theory, these sachets are just what we want, but in practice we will see that using them has certain, often serious, drawbacks that overshadow their advantages.

The advantages and disadvantages of powdered proteins

- The advantages. For a long time the laboratories that sold powdered proteins promoted their purity as their main advantage. In fact, this advantage is insignificant. During my programme's first two phases and until the True Weight is reached, the absolute purity of these powders has no decisive advantage over protein foods, neither as far as length of time or weight loss are concerned. In permanent stabilization, when the diet is only for one day a week, there is some sense in using them to strengthen the impact of protein Thursdays but here again they are far from indispensable.

   Powdered proteins also have the advantage of being clean, easy to carry around and practical to use in any busy work situation, if you have irregular hours and no time to prepare food or eat at regular mealtimes.

- The disadvantages. The first and main drawback of powdered proteins is that they are artificial. A human being is not biologically programmed to eat powder. All our senses – sight, touch, smell, taste – as well as those parts of the brain which control our feelings of satisfaction and pleasure, make us choose to feed ourselves with foods that have a particular appearance, flavour, aroma and texture: quite simply human foods! And when I say human, this is not just an empty word or intellectual, philosophical or moral posturing; I am talking about effectiveness. Now is a good time to briefly give you my analysis of the reasons for

155

the current weight crisis, based on my 40 years of experience and work in the field.

Yes, we are putting on weight because we eat too much and take too little exercise. But what exactly are we saying? In Western societies, we all face both the same abundance of foods and the same temptation to be sedentary. So why is it, for example, that 40 million French people manage not to become overweight whereas the other 20 million get stuck? Yes, we know how we put on weight; all that matters is to understand why. Why do a third of all French people eat too much and exercise too little while at the same time hating it?

Well, perhaps I am going to surprise you but this is what I truly believe having seen it every day and with practically every patient who comes to me for a consultation. Twenty million French people put on weight because they are unable to adapt to the invisible but very real difficulty of our current way of life. A way of life that is fast, rich and comfortable but which no longer offers this large group of people a sufficient dose of pleasure, contentment and self-fulfilment. This may be temporary or long-standing, linked to the economic climate or the way our society is, but it affects the quality of our day-to-day life and food offers an extremely effective outlet for frustration. And the loss of what is natural, instinctive and human contributes to this dissatisfaction and difficulty in adapting to modern life. So here we are back again with these powders that offer us more artificiality and in the very realm of food, a realm that is both the most fundamentally instinctive and whose emotional charge is matched only by orgasm.

A white or pale powder, even when sweetened and flavoured, does not have any of the stimuli that really satisfy us. Feeding ourselves does consist in swallowing a certain quantity of energy and nutrients. It also fulfils our very basic need for pleasure, which we achieve by satisfying our instincts and sensory organs. This is increasingly true as we compensate for the stresses modern life imposes on us.

Nutritionists have learnt to their cost that prolonged use of powdered-protein diets by young and vulnerable people can result in bulimia, causing instability that makes any hope of stabilization impossible. For this profound and fundamental reason, this type of food must be limited to only occasional use.

- I will only briefly mention the other drawbacks as they are technical and just apply to those who are real enthusiasts for these powders, mostly novices who are convinced by the advertising that they will lose weight really quickly. This is true but they will put it back on again even more quickly having upset their ponderostat – the weight-control centre located in the brain – forever. Firstly, the price: slimming with sachets is very expensive. Secondly, their purity and their quality are not always comparable. Avoid vegetable proteins as they are often incomplete and stick with milk or egg white proteins. Moreover, powdered proteins should not be confused with powdered meal substitutes whose ratios of proteins, lipids and glucose are just the same as any traditional meal, but lacking the pleasure of real food. Finally, their total lack of fibre, which causes serious constipation.

To conclude, if you want to lose weight and use them over a prolonged period, powdered proteins have absolutely nothing to offer besides a considerable number of drawbacks – and very serious ones at that. Used once or occasionally, they can prove handy to avoid skipping a meal or replace something even more dangerous, a high-risk meal or a fast-food sandwich.

Do Not Take Lifts or Escalators

This instruction is an integral part of my stabilization programme. Anyone, especially someone who has lost many pounds and knows how much effort this has cost and how much satisfaction it has given them, has to accept this extremely simple pledge, which is to give up using lifts and escalators. At a time when expensive step machines are sold and gym subscriptions make a hole in many people's pockets, why not think of the stairs as a little exercise you can include for free in your normal daily activities. Here again, you see this advice bandied around like a handy magazine tip; I make a habit of writing it out at the top on my prescriptions and I have noticed that this is far more effective.

Going up or down the stairs makes the body's largest muscles contract and, in a short time, uses up a considerable number of calories. Moreover, it gets sedentary city folk to change their heartbeat regularly, which is an excellent way of preventing coronaries. However, as well as getting you into the habit of burning up calories in the long term this instruction also has a deeper purpose. It allows you several times a day to test your determination to never put weight on again.

At the bottom of the stairs, equidistant between the lift and the first steps, anyone trying to stabilize their weight is symbolically confronted with a choice that helps them measure their determination. Grabbing hold of the banister and walking up enthusiastically is a simple, practical and logical choice, a kind of wink from my reader to tell me that they believe in my programme, that they are following it and that it works for them.

Choosing the lift or escalator with the excuse that you are late or your shopping is too heavy is a sign that you are letting go and that this is just the beginning. A stabilization programme where you are unwilling to make a modest contribution is doomed to failure. So always firmly opt for the stairs.

Stabilizing Fibre: Three Tablespoons of Oat Bran Every Day for Life

In the first part of the book I have already looked at oat bran in some detail and I think I have covered everything, but I will just add an observation from my experience as a nutritionist. I have noticed that the patients, readers and internet users from my coaching website who have achieved the best results and stabilization in the long term are those who most regularly eat bran and in particular the galettes, which they make a habit of eating twice a day, one in the morning and one in the middle of the afternoon.

I think that in addition to its nutritional effects, making you lose calories and feel full, just like taking the stairs and pure protein Thursdays, oat bran stands guard over you, making sure that you are still on course, aware of any dangers and equipped to deal with them.

In practice, you now have to include your three tablespoons in your daily routine. There is nothing to stop you having a fourth if one day you feel the need or inclination.

A small precaution

In so far as oat bran slows down the assimilation of nutrients, causing loss from the intestinal bolus, I am often asked if it does the same with vitamins and certain medications. The answer is yes. But only to a small extent as vitamins and medication are present in tiny quantities. There is nothing to fear with a dose of up to three tablespoons. However, I have noted that some patients can easily exceed this dose, in which case it is best to take a multivitamin supplement and, if you need special medication, to wait for one hour after eating the oat bran (I repeat this is only if you are taking more than the three tablespoons).

Permanent Stabilization Diet Summary

1. Go back to eating what you want six days out of seven, while keeping the consolidation foods as your safety base and platform.
2. Hold on to everything you have learnt and the good habits you have acquired while completing the whole programme.
3. Enshrine protein Thursdays as the day that protects you for the rest of your life.
4. Live your life as if lifts and escalators did not exist.
5. Also, take three tablespoons of oat bran every day for the rest of your life.

If you neglect any of these five measures you will put your weight management at risk. If you give them all up, sooner or later you will definitely put back on all the weight you have lost.

RECIPES AND MENUS

The pure protein diet, which is the spearhead of the weight-loss part of my programme and stabilization Thursdays, should be familiar to you by now. If you have already started, then you have probably noticed its surprising mixture of effectiveness and simplicity. One of the best things about the Dukan Diet is this simplicity, which eliminates all ambiguity by focusing on exactly which foods you can eat. But this diet also has its Achilles heel. Some patients, because they lack time or imagination, limit themselves to a repertoire of steaks, crab sticks, extra-lean hams, hard-boiled eggs and non-fat yoghurt, repeating the same menu day after day.

This solution is of course in line with the diet's creed, which is to allow you to eat freely within the list of permitted foods. But, eventually, limiting yourself in this way becomes monotonous and wearisome, wrongly creating the impression that this diet lacks variety.

But it does not, so it is absolutely essential, especially for anyone who has a lot of weight to lose, to make a bit of an effort to ensure that this diet is not only bearable, but actually appetizing and attractive.

From my consultations, I have seen that given the list of permitted foods certain people are more inventive than others and manage to create bold dishes and combinations, as well as innovative recipes that make their diet enjoyable. I started writing down these recipes and giving them to other patients who had less time or creativity, instigating a recipe exchange for anyone about to start the Dukan Diet.

These recipes strictly use the list of foods for the protein Attack diet and then the list for the Cruise diet with its protein foods and vegetables. They are only suggestions and in no way prevent inventive readers from coming up with original ideas to make every day even more varied.

The ultimate purpose of this recipe collection is to save time so that anyone using them can spend more on improving the quality and presentation of their dishes and meals.

Sauces, Mayonnaise and Dressings

The vast majority of sauces require large quantities of oil, butter or cream, which are the chief enemies of anyone wanting to lose weight. For this reason these ingredients are excluded from the first two phases of the Dukan Diet, which are strictly about losing weight. The one exception is tiny, almost negligible amounts of vegetable oil (of your choice) when necessary, including the one teaspoon in Vinaigrette Maya.

The major problem in following my programme and in particular its first two phases is therefore finding suitable sauces and seasonings to accompany some noble foods such as meat, fish, eggs and poultry.

We can replace fats with several available alternatives, including the following:

- Guar gum. This little-known vegetable ingredient is sold in powder form. Containing virtually no calories, its natural gel-like qualities mean that it can be used to thicken sauces and dressings, giving them a creamy, smooth texture similar to oil-based sauces. Just a tiny amount, ¼ teaspoon for 150ml (5fl oz) of liquid, is enough to thicken sauces when heated.
- Cornflour. This ingredient, a cousin of tapioca, is useful for its thickening and binding properties. Although it is a carbohydrate, you need such tiny amounts, 1 teaspoon for 125ml (4fl oz) of sauce, that it is allowed. Cornflour, like guar gum, makes sauces, especially béchamel, creamy without adding any fat.

  Before you use it, you must thin it with a small amount of cold liquid – water, milk or bouillon – before you add it to the hot mixture. It thickens when heated.
- Low-fat bouillon cubes (beef, chicken, fish and vegetable). These are very useful for certain sauces, not just for their thickening and binding qualities when replacing oil in salad dressings, but also when mixed with a bed of chopped sautéed onions to accompany meat and fish, to add flavour without fat.

I now suggest a few recipes for some basic sauces and dressings using these ingredients.

Vinaignette is a basic, but important, dressing for the Cruise phase, so that you can enjoy salads and raw vegetables; it can be adapted to suit all tastes.

VINAIGRETTE MAYA

1 tablespoon Dijon mustard or Meaux à l'ancienne
5 tablespoons balsamic vinegar
1 teaspoon vegetable oil
1 garlic clove
7–8 fresh or frozen chopped basil leaves
Salt and black pepper

Take an old mustard jar and fill it with all the ingredients, mixing very thoroughly. If you like garlic, leave a clove to marinate in the bottom of the jar.

VEGETABLE BOUILLON VINAIGRETTE

1 low-fat vegetable bouillon cube
2 tablespoons hot water
1 level teaspoon cornflour
2 tablespoons vinegar
1 tablespoon French Meaux à l'ancienne

Dilute the bouillon cube in hot water, add the cornflour, vinegar and mustard, and mix together well.

DUKAN HERB MAYONNAISE

1 raw egg yolk
1 tablespoon Dijon mustard
3 tablespoons non-fat fromage frais or quark
1 tablespoon chopped parsley or chives
Salt and black pepper

Put the egg yolk in a mixing bowl and combine with the mustard. Season with salt and pepper and add the herbs. Gradually mix in the fromage frais or quark, stirring continuously. Mayonnaise must be refrigerated.

ALTERNATIVE OIL-FREE MAYONNAISE

1 hard-boiled egg
55g (2oz) non-fat fromage frais or quark
½ teaspoon Dijon mustard
Salt and black pepper

Crush the hard-boiled egg with a fork and mix into the non-fat fromage frais or quark. Then add the mustard, salt and pepper, and some herbs if you wish. Mayonnaise must be refrigerated.

SAUCE BÉARNAISE DE REGIME
(DIET BÉARNAISE SAUCE)

2 teaspoons white vinegar
1 small shallot, finely chopped
¼ teaspoon tarragon, crushed or chopped according
   to taste
2 egg yolks

Put the vinegar in a bowl in a saucepan over simmering water, then add the chopped shallot and tarragon. Slowly warm over a low heat. Let the vinegar mixture cool, then pour it over the two egg yolks, beating well as if making mayonnaise.

SAUCE RAVIGOTE ('RAVIGOTE' SAUCE)

1 hard-boiled egg
3 medium-size gherkins, finely diced
1 small onion, chopped
2 tablespoons each of chopped chives, parsley
  and tarragon
2 small pots non-fat yoghurt
½ teaspoon Dijon mustard
Salt

In a glass bowl mix together the egg, gherkins, onion and herbs. Add the yoghurt, mustard and salt. Serve with fish, hard-boiled eggs, meat and vegetables.

SAUCE BLANCHE (WHITE SAUCE)

125ml (4fl oz) skimmed milk
2 egg yolks, beaten
1 small pot non-fat yoghurt
Salt and black pepper

In a double saucepan, heat the milk until lukewarm then add salt and pepper. Pour a small amount of the milk over the egg yolks, then incorporate the eggs and milk mixture into the pan. Beat well and add the yoghurt. Heat the sauce through. If serving with fish you can add some chopped gherkin.

COULIS DE TOMATES (TOMATO SAUCE)

70g (2½ oz) finely chopped onion
6–8 fresh tomatoes, peeled and seeds removed
    (or 1 x 410g (14½oz) can peeled tomatoes)
½ teaspoon basil
½ teaspoon fresh mint
½ teaspoon tarragon
Salt and black pepper

Put the chopped onion and fresh (or canned) tomatoes in a non-stick saucepan, add salt and pepper to taste. Cover and simmer over a low heat for 20 minutes. Let the sauce cool then add the herbs. Serve with fish and vegetables in the cruising stage.

SAUCE AUX FINES HERBES (HERB SAUCE)

1 low-fat bouillon cube (meat, fish or vegetable)
1 teaspoon cornflour
200g (7oz) non-fat fromage frais or quark
Herbs (watercress, parsley, tarragon, chives, mint or
    small shallots)
Salt and black pepper

Dissolve a bouillon cube in half a glass of lukewarm water and slowly add the cornflour, mixing all the time. Place in a saucepan over a low heat and stir until it thickens. Remove from the heat and mix in the non-fat fromage frais or quark, herbs, and salt and pepper to taste. Serve with either fish or meat.

SAUCE CHASSEUR (HUNTER'S SAUCE)

2 finely chopped shallots
3 tablespoons vinegar
2 tablespoons water
1 beaten egg yolk
2 tablespoons non-fat fromage frais or quark
1 sprig tarragon, chopped
Salt and black pepper

In a saucepan, mix the chopped shallots with the vinegar and water. Cover and cook for about 10 minutes. Uncover and continue cooking until the sauce thickens, for 5 more minutes. Remove from the heat, add the beaten egg yolk and quark or fromage frais. Then add the chopped tarragon and season to taste. Reheat in a double saucepan to thicken further. Serve with meat and fish.

SAUCE HOLLANDAISE (HOLLANDAISE SAUCE)

1 egg yolk
1 teaspoon Dijon mustard
2 tablespoons lemon juice
50ml (2fl oz) warm skimmed milk

Combine the egg yolk, mustard and lemon juice in a double saucepan over simmering but not boiling water. Let this heat for a few minutes to thicken and then, stirring slowly, add the warm milk. Let the sauce thicken, and keep warm until needed. Serve with white fish, asparagus, French beans and spinach in the cruising stage.

SAUCE BÉCHAMEL (BÉCHAMEL SAUCE)

250ml (9fl oz) cold skimmed milk
1 tablespoon cornflour
1 low-fat beef bouillon cube
Salt, black pepper and nutmeg

In a saucepan, mix together the cold milk and cornflour, then add the bouillon cube. Let this cook for a few minutes on a low heat until it thickens. Add salt, pepper and nutmeg to taste. Ideal for vegetable gratins and chicory wrapped in ham during the cruising stage.

SAUCE AU RAIFORT (HORSERADISH SAUCE)

225ml (8fl oz) non-fat fromage frais or quark
1 tablespoon chopped horseradish
Salt and black pepper

Mix the fromage frais or quark with the horseradish, salt and pepper until a fine, light mixture is obtained. Serve with fish that has been steamed, microwaved or cooked 'en papillote'. Also good with white meats, such as pork and poultry.

SAUCE DIVINE (HEAVENLY SAUCE)

2 egg yolks
1 tablespoon Dijon mustard
150g (5½oz) non-fat fromage frais or quark
1 teaspoon cornflour
Chopped herbs (dill, parsley, tarragon, etc.)
Fresh lemon juice
Salt and black pepper

In a saucepan mix together the egg yolks, mustard, fromage frais or quark and cornflour. Season to taste. Gently bring to the boil. Remove from the heat and add some chopped herbs and lemon juice. Serve hot or warm with cooked fish.

Meat Recipes for the Attack Diet

RÔTI DE BOEUF (ROAST BEEF)
(4–6 servings)

You will need a meat thermometer.

1.3kg (3lb) sirloin or fillet of beef
Salt and black pepper

Preheat the oven to 240°C/475°F/Gas 9.
Roast the beef in a dish, uncovered, for 15 minutes. Do not add salt until after it is cooked so that the juices do not dry out. Reduce the oven temperature to 160°C/325°F/Gas 3. Continue to roast until the thermometer inserted into the centre of the roast shows 49°C/120°F, another 35–45 minutes. Transfer the roast to a chopping board and let it stand, uncovered, for 15 minutes. Season to taste, then carve and serve.

Cold beef leftovers: Serve using one of the many sauces described on the previous pages.

BROCHETTES DE FILET DE BOEUF (BEEF KEBABS)

(4 servings)

You will need 4 skewers.

400g (14oz) beef fillet, cut into large chunks
50ml (2fl oz) low-sodium soy sauce
2 tablespoons Dijon mustard
1 tablespoon cider vinegar
A little thyme
1 bay leaf
A dash of vegetable oil
50ml (2fl oz) fresh lemon juice

Mix all the ingredients together and marinate the beef for 2–4 hours in the refrigerator. Discard the marinade. Place the chunks of beef on the skewers (if using wooden skewers, make sure you soak them in water first to prevent them burning). Grill until cooked to your liking.

During the Cruise phase you may add tomatoes, mushrooms, peppers and onions to the skewer. During the Attack phase you can add these for the taste they give the meat and to make the kebabs look attractive but do not eat the vegetables.

STEAK AU POIVRE (PEPPER STEAK)

(4 servings)

600g (1¼lb) good sirloin steak (about 2–2.5cm/
¾–1in thick)
1 small pot non-fat yoghurt
1 teaspoon vegetable oil
Freshly ground black pepper

Cook the steak in a non-stick frying pan, then cover with coarsely ground black pepper. In another saucepan, warm the yoghurt. Add the vegetable oil and season with pepper. Pour half this mixture on to the steak when it is still very hot. Turn off the heat, but leave the steak in the pan. Stir the rest of the sauce, pour over the steak and serve.

BOEUF BOUILLI (BOILED BEEF)

(4 servings)

450g (1lb) lean sirloin
1.5 litres (2½ pints) water
1 teaspoon thyme
1 bay leaf
1 low-fat beef bouillon cube
1 onion
Salt and black pepper
Gherkins, to serve

Put the meat, water, thyme, bay leaf, bouillon cube, onion, salt and pepper in a large pot. Cook for 1 hour and 15 minutes on a medium heat. Cool until lukewarm then cut into cubes. Serve with *Sauce Ravigote* (see page 168) and gherkins.

In the Cruise phase, add a leek to the stew. Serve with tomato sauce.

RÔTI DE BOEUF HACHÉ (MEAT LOAF)
(makes enough for 10–12 slices)

1.2 kg (2½lb) lean minced beef
1 finely chopped onion
2 eggs, beaten
4 tablespoons non-fat fromage frais or yoghurt
2 hard-boiled eggs, sliced
Salt and black pepper

Preheat the oven to 180°C/350°F/Gas 4.

Carefully mix the chopped onion, beaten eggs, fromage frais or yoghurt, salt and pepper into the minced beef. Lightly oil and dust with flour a bread tin, then add half the mixture. Place the sliced hard-boiled eggs on top in a row then add the rest of the meatloaf mixture. Cook for 1 hour. Let the loaf stand for 10 minutes before slicing. Serve hot or cold with the *Sauce au Raifort* (see page 171), *Sauce aux Fines Herbes* (see page 169) or *Coulis de Tomates* (see page 169) in the Cruise phase.

BOEUF LUC LAC (LUC LAC BEEF)

(2 servings)

400g (14oz) beef
2 tablespoons soy sauce
1 tablespoon oyster sauce
1 large piece ginger, crushed
4 garlic cloves, crushed
A few coriander leaves, to garnish
Black pepper

Cut the meat into 1cm (½in) cubes and season with the soy sauce, oyster sauce, crushed ginger and pepper. Leave to marinate for at least 30 minutes. Just before you are ready to serve, grease a frying pan with a drop of vegetable oil and gently fry the garlic. Once the garlic has started to brown and smell good, add the meat and cook over a very high heat. Mix together rapidly for 10–15 seconds. The meat should still be a little rare so do not overcook. Garnish with a few fresh coriander leaves.

ESCALOPE DE VEAU (VEAL MEDALLIONS)

(4 servings)

450g (1lb) lean, trimmed veal
1 small onion, sliced (used only for flavour)
1 garlic clove, crushed
1 low-fat bouillon cube, dissolved in 2 tablespoons
  water

1 lemon, cut into quarters
Salt and black pepper

Pound the veal between sheets of plastic wrap until 3mm ($\frac{1}{8}$in) thick, then cut into 16 equal pieces. Sprinkle with salt and pepper. Prepare a bed of onions and garlic in a non-stick frying pan and sprinkle over the bouillon liquid. Cook until the onions caramelize. Place the veal medallions on the bed of onions and cook for 10 minutes on each side. Remove the onions and quickly cook the meat over a high heat in the remaining juices. Serve with fresh lemon wedges.

CÔTE DE VEAU POÊLÉE (SAUTÉED VEAL CHOPS)

(4 servings)

4 lean veal chops
1 small onion, sliced (used only for flavour)
1 garlic clove, crushed
1 low-fat bouillon cube, dissolved in 2 tablespoons water
1 lemon, cut into quarters
2 gherkins, sliced
Salt and black pepper

Sprinkle the veal chops with salt and pepper. Prepare a bed of onions and garlic in a non-stick frying pan and sprinkle over the bouillon liquid. Cook until the onions caramelize. Put the veal chops on the bed of onions, cook for 10 minutes on each side then add 2 tablespoons water and cook for another minute. Remove the onions and turn the meat over a high heat in the remaining juices. Serve with fresh lemon wedges and gherkin slices.

FOIE DE VEAU POÊLÉ AU VINAIGRE DE XÉRÈES (VEAL LIVER SAUTÉED IN SHERRY VINEGAR)

(2 servings, can be doubled)

350g (12oz) veal's liver
1 small onion, sliced or chopped
1 large garlic clove, crushed
1 teaspoon fresh lemon juice
1½ tablespoons sherry vinegar

Put the onion and garlic in a non-stick frying pan and slowly cook on a medium heat until they caramelize. Place the liver on top of the onions and cook for 6–10 minutes on each side. Remove the onions, then add the lemon juice and vinegar to the juices and cook the liver on a high heat until done.

LANGUE DE BOEUF SAUCE RAVIGOTE (BEEF TONGUE WITH 'RAVIGOTE' SAUCE)

(4 servings)

1 beef tongue, trimmed of fat
1.5 litres (2½ pints) water
1 teaspoon thyme
1 bay leaf
1 whole onion
Salt and black pepper

Place the tongue, water, thyme, bay leaf, onion, salt and black pepper in a large pot. Cook for 1 hour and 15 minutes on a medium heat. Cut into slices and serve warm, with *Sauce Ravigote* (see page 168) and pickles. Remember to use only the front part of the tongue – the leanest part is closest to the tip.

Poultry Recipes for the Attack Diet

POULET À L'ESTRAGON (ROAST CHICKEN WITH TARRAGON AND LEMON)

(6 servings)

1 roasting chicken, washed, rinsed and patted dry
*   with kitchen paper*
1 garlic clove, diced
Fresh tarragon
1 fresh lemon, cut in half

1 whole onion
Salt and black pepper

Preheat the oven to 220°C/425°F/Gas 7.
Rub the chicken with the garlic, some fresh tarragon and a lemon half. Chop the remaining tarragon and place it inside the chicken with the onion and other lemon half. Cover with foil and cook in the oven until the juices run clear. Remove the foil and let the top brown for the last 10 minutes. Avoid eating the skin and the tips of the wings.

SOUFFLÉ DE POULET (CHICKEN SOUFFLÉ)

(4 servings)

115g (4oz) white chicken meat, in bite-size pieces
A sprinkling of dried herbs (thyme, rosemary, sage
*   and nutmeg)*
225ml (8fl oz) skimmed milk
2 eggs, separated – egg whites at room temperature
Salt and black pepper

Preheat the oven to 160°C/325°F/Gas 3.
Lightly oil and dust a 1.2 litre (2 pint) soufflé dish. Mix together the chicken, salt, pepper and herbs. Heat up the skimmed milk and pour it over the two egg yolks. Mix the milk and egg mixture with the chopped chicken and herbs and put into the soufflé dish. Whip the egg whites until soft peaks form (do not overbeat).

Carefully fold them into the chicken mixture (so that the soufflé will rise). Cook in a medium hot oven for a good half hour. Serve immediately.

POULET MOUTARDE
(CHICKEN WITH MUSTARD)

(4 servings)

8 skinless chicken thighs with bones
115g (4oz) Dijon mustard
1 teaspoon thyme
1 teaspoon vegetable oil
175g (6oz) non-fat yoghurt or fromage frais
Salt and black pepper
Gherkin slices, to serve

Preheat the oven to 200°C/400°F/Gas 6.
Place a sheet of aluminium foil on a large baking sheet and on it put the chicken thighs coated with mustard and sprinkled with thyme. Place another piece of aluminium foil over the first, to make a pouch. Seal the foil seams completely so that no steam can escape. Put in the preheated oven and cook for 45–60 minutes. When the chicken is almost cooked, mix together the oil and non-fat yoghurt or fromage frais, and season with salt and pepper. Continue baking the chicken until done. Remove the foil and pour the sauce over the chicken thighs, dissolving the dried mustard. Serve with gherkin slices.

ESCALOPES DE POULET TANDOORI
(TANDOORI CHICKEN ESCALOPES)

(6 servings)

6 chicken breast fillets
2 small pots non-fat yoghurt
2 tablespoons tandoori masala spice mix
3 garlic cloves, crushed
2cm (¾in) piece ginger, crushed
2 green chillies, crushed
Lemon juice
Salt and black pepper

Mix all the ingredients together, except the meat. Make sure that the garlic, ginger, chillies and spices are completely crushed to make a smooth blend. Score the chicken so that the yoghurt-spice mixture gets right inside the meat and leave to marinate overnight in the fridge. The next day cook in a moderate oven – 200°C/400°F/Gas 6 – for 20 minutes then brown under the grill before serving.

POULET À L'INDIENNE (INDIAN CHICKEN)

(4 servings)

1 whole chicken, cut into pieces
1 lemon
3 small pots non-fat yoghurt
4 tablespoons chopped ginger

3 garlic cloves, chopped
1 teaspoon cinnamon
2 pinches Cayenne chilli pepper
1 teaspoon coriander seeds
3 cloves
10 mint leaves, chopped
2 onions, finely chopped
1 tablespoon water
1 low-fat chicken bouillon cube
Salt and black pepper

Zest the lemon. In a bowl mix together the yoghurt, ginger, garlic, spices, lemon zest and mint leaves. Season the chicken pieces, add to the yoghurt mixture and leave to marinate in the fridge for 24 hours. The following day brown the onions in a non-stick casserole dish with the water then add the chicken and marinade. Simmer over a gentle heat for about 1 hour. Make soup with the remaining juices by adding a low-fat chicken bouillon cube. Serve hot.

POULET AU CITRON (LEMON CHICKEN)
(2 servings)

500g (1lb 2oz) chicken
1 onion, thinly sliced
2 garlic cloves, chopped
½ teaspoon finely chopped ginger
Juice and zest of 2 lemons

2 tablespoons soy sauce
1 bouquet garni
1 pinch cinnamon
1 pinch powdered ginger
Salt and black pepper

Cut the meat into medium-size cubes. In a non-stick casserole dish gently fry the onion, garlic and ginger over a moderate heat for 3–4 minutes. Add the meat and stir for 2 minutes with a spatula to brown over a high heat. Moisten with the lemon juice, soy sauce and 150ml (¼ pint) water. Add the bouquet garni, cinnamon, powdered ginger and lemon zest. Then season with salt and pepper and simmer, covered, over a gentle heat for 45 minutes. Serve hot.

Fish and Seafood Recipes for the Attack Diet

SOLE NATURE CUITE VAPEUR (STEAMED SOLE)
(4 servings)

Note: this fish is steamed on plates so it holds the juices around the fillets.

900g (2lb) sole fillets, cut into 8 pieces
2 tablespoons chopped parsley
1 lemon, cut into quarters
Salt and black pepper

Wash and pat dry the fillets with kitchen towel. Transfer the fish between 2 rimmed plates (make sure there is a large enough rim to cover the edges of the saucepan). Fill a saucepan three-quarters full of water. Bring the water to the boil. Put the plates of fish on top of the pan, with the rims resting on the edges. The fish will be perfectly cooked in 15 minutes. Garnish with the chopped parsley, and season. Serve immediately with the lemon wedges.

POISSON SAUCE BLANCHE (WHITE FISH WITH WHITE SAUCE)

(4 servings)

4 x 175g (6oz) hake, halibut or cod steaks
850ml (1½ pints) water
10 whole peppercorns
1 shallot, chopped
1 low-fat vegetable bouillon cube
2 bay leaves

Bring the water, peppercorns, shallot, bouillon cube and bay leaves to boiling point in a deep poaching pan over a medium heat. Reduce to a simmer and add the fish. Poach, uncovered, until opaque and cooked through – about 6 minutes. Discard the pan juices. Serve with *Sauce Blanche* (see page 168).

DAURADE ROYALE (SEA BREAM ROYAL)

(4 servings)

*4 x 140g (5oz) skinless sea bream fillets (2cm/¾in thick),
   bones removed*
450g (1lb) fresh mussels, rinsed and well scrubbed
1 large onion, sliced
125ml (4fl oz) dry white wine
Lemon juice
Salt and black pepper
Lemon wedges, to serve

Preheat the oven to 230°C/450°F/Gas 8.

Wash the fish fillets carefully, then place them in a large baking dish and garnish with the sliced onion. In a large saucepan, steam the mussels in the wine over a medium heat until they open. Discard any unopened mussels. Take the juice from the mussels, add the lemon juice and strain it well. Pour this liquid over the sea bream and season with freshly grated black pepper. Put the fish into the oven and cook, uncovered, for 30 minutes until done. Shell the mussels and add them to the fish for the last 5 minutes of cooking time with 2 tablespoons water and a pinch of salt. Discard the juices from the pan and serve with fresh lemon wedges.

DAURADE GRILLÉE (GRILLED SEA BREAM)

(4 servings)

4 x 140g (5oz) boneless sea bream fillets
¼ teaspoon dill
¼ teaspoon tarragon
½ small onion, chopped
Salt and black pepper
Lemon wedges, to serve

Wash and pat dry the fillets with kitchen towel. Sprinkle on the herbs and onion, and season with pepper. Place the fish either on the grill (with the rack lightly oiled with vegetable oil so the fish doesn't stick), or in a moderate oven until it is done – about 20 minutes. Add salt after cooking. Serve with fresh lemon wedges.

SAUMON EN PAPILLOTE (BAKED SALMON PARCEL)

(4 servings)

4 x 175g (6oz) salmon steaks from the middle
of the fish
1 teaspoon dill
1 lemon, squeezed
1 leek, sliced and 1 onion, sliced (for flavour only; will
be discarded for the Attack diet)
Salt and black pepper

Preheat the oven to 200°C/400°F/Gas 6.

Place the salmon on aluminium foil on a baking sheet, leaving enough extra foil to make a pouch. Sprinkle with the dill, lemon juice, salt and pepper. Add the onion and leek slices for flavouring (to be discarded after cooking). Tightly seal the foil seams to preserve the salmon's texture and the rich flavours in the juice. Cook for 20 minutes, or less, according to your taste. Serve immediately.

SAUMON GRILLÉ À L'UNILATÉRALE (GRILLED SALMON)

(4 servings)

4 x 175g (6oz) salmon steaks from the centre
Salt and black pepper
Fresh dill, to garnish
Lemon wedges, to serve

Place the salmon, skin side up, on a baking dish or sheet covered with aluminium foil and liberally sprinkle with coarse salt. Cook under the grill until the salt is wet with juice and the skin begins to brown and crack. At this point, the meat just under the skin is cooked, firm and a bright orange colour. Remove the salmon, scrape off the salt and turn it over. Salmon is best when it is just cooked to perfection, not overcooked, still with its salmon colour, steamy hot on the skin side, and just warm but nicely pink on the surface. Garnish with dill and serve with fresh lemon wedges. Use up any leftover salmon served cold with *Dukan Herb Mayonnaise* (see page 166).

SAUMON AU FOUR (BAKED SALMON)

(4 servings)

4 x 175g (6oz) salmon fillets from the centre
125ml (4fl oz) dry white wine
4 fresh sprigs of dill
Salt and black pepper
Lemon wedges, to serve

Preheat the oven to 190°C/375°F/Gas 5.
Wash and pat dry the fish. Place the fish skin side down in a clear baking dish. Add the wine and some black pepper. Put the sprigs of dill on each fillet. Bake until just opaque in the centre, about 20 minutes. Lightly salt, and discard the pan juices. Serve with fresh lemon wedges.

SAUMON POCHÉ (POACHED SALMON FILLETS)

(6 servings)

6 x 175g (6oz) salmon fillets from the centre
100ml (3½fl oz) water
100ml (3½fl oz) dry white wine
1 shallot, finely sliced

4 sprigs of parsley
Thyme
Lemon wedges, to serve

Combine the water, wine, shallot, parsley and thyme in a large poaching pan. Add the salmon fillets, skin side down. Cover tightly and simmer on a medium heat for about 10 minutes. Remove from the heat and allow to stand for 5 minutes. Discard the pan juices and serve with fresh lemon wedges. Leftover salmon can be served cold with Dukan Herb Mayonnaise (see page 166).

SAUMON CRU MARINÉ
(MARINATED RAW SALMON)

(4 servings)

675g (1½lb) smoked salmon
Juice of 1 lemon
¼ teaspoon dill
¼ teaspoon tarragon
1 green pepper, de-seeded and sliced (for flavour only)
Salt and black pepper

Place the salmon in a shallow baking dish. Sprinkle with the lemon, dill and tarragon, salt and black pepper. Add the green pepper, then leave to marinate and chill overnight. Discard the pepper. Cut into slices, decorate with dill and serve.

TARTARE DE SAUMON (SALMON TARTAR)

(2 servings)

225g (½lb) smoked salmon, chopped
155ml (4fl oz) Sauce aux Fines Herbes (see page 169)

Mix the chopped salmon and herb sauce together thoroughly, ensuring they are well blended. Add more sauce to suit your own preference.

MOULES MARINIÈRES

(2 servings, can be doubled)

900g (2lb) medium-size mussels, scrubbed
*   and rinsed several times*
½ medium onion, sliced
2 garlic cloves, chopped
¼ teaspoon thyme
1 bay leaf
225ml (8fl oz) dry white wine
¼ teaspoon ground black pepper
55g (2oz) chopped parsley
¼ teaspoon salt

Place the cleaned mussels in a pot with all the ingredients listed above except the salt. Cover the pot and cook over a high heat. Shake the pot until the mussels open up, 4–5 minutes. Discard any unopened ones. Put them on a platter with the lightly salted juice and serve.

RAMEQUINS DE MOULES (BAKED MUSSELS)

(4 servings)

2kg (4lb 8oz) mussels, scrubbed and rinsed well
225ml (8fl oz) dry white wine
3 eggs
1 tablespoon non-fat fromage frais or quark,
   thinned with water
30g (1oz) parsley, chopped
Salt and black pepper

Preheat the oven to 230°C/450°F/Gas 8.
Put the mussels in a large saucepan with the white wine and steam on a high heat until they open, shaking the pan occasionally. Discard any that do not open. Shake the mussels and drain off the liquid into a strainer. While the liquid is still warm mix in the eggs, fromage frais or quark and parsley. Season. Place the mussels in individual ramekins or a large soufflé dish and cook in the oven for 10 minutes. Serve immediately.

CRABE FARCI (STUFFED CRAB)

(4 servings)

675g (1½lb) fresh crabmeat (cartilage removed)
Mayonnaise (see page 167)
4 hard-boiled eggs, peeled and sliced

Mix together the mayonnaise and crabmeat and serve with slices of hard-boiled egg. For the Cruise diet, add sliced tomatoes and salad leaves.

COQUILLES SAINT-JACQUES EN GRATIN (SCALLOPS GRATIN)

(4 servings)

4 large scallops
450g (1lb) mussels, scrubbed and rinsed
115g (4oz) shrimps, peeled, de-veined and rinsed
1 litre (1¾ pints) water
3 tablespoons wine vinegar
50ml (2fl oz) dry white wine
2 hard-boiled eggs, mashed
1 shallot, chopped
15g (½oz) fresh parsley, chopped or 1 tablespoon if dry

Preheat the oven to 200°C/400°F/Gas 6.
Cook the scallops for 15 minutes in a saucepan with the water and vinegar. Cook the mussels over a high heat with the wine until they are completely open (discard

any unopened ones). Strain the liquid. Mix together the eggs, shallot and parsley, then add the shelled mussels and shrimps. Cut the scallops into large cubes and add them to the mixture. To moisten, add some juice from the mussels until you have a rich, smooth blend. Divide the mixture into 4 ramekins and place them on a baking sheet in the oven. Bake for 20–25 minutes.

LANGOUSTINES MAYONNAISE
(SCAMPI WITH MAYONNAISE)

(2 servings, can be doubled)

900g (2lb) scampi, peeled, de-veined and rinsed
1 litre (1¾ pints) water
3 tablespoons vinegar
Mayonnaise (see page 167)

Put the scampi in boiling water with the vinegar, cook until pink, then let them cool in the water. Serve with mayonnaise.

CREVETTES AUX HERBES
(SHRIMPS SAUTÉED IN HERBS)

(2 servings, can be doubled)

900g (2lb) shrimps, peeled, de-veined and rinsed
4 garlic cloves, crushed
30g (1oz) parsley, chopped

50ml (2fl oz) dry white wine
1 lemon, cut in half

In a non-stick frying pan add the shrimps, garlic, parsley and wine. Sauté on a medium heat until the shrimps are pink. Serve with fresh lemon.

PLATEAU DE FRUITS DE MER (SEAFOOD PLATTER)

(8 servings)

12 fresh oysters, rinsed and prepared
900g (2lb) mussels, steamed
900g (2lb) shrimps, rinsed and cooked
900g (2lb) clams, steamed
Lemon wedges, to serve

Steam the mussels, shrimps and clams separately. Cool completely. Arrange all the seafood with the oysters in their half shells on a platter with a bed of crushed ice decorated with seaweed. Serve with fresh lemon wedges.

Egg Recipes for the Attack Diet

Eggs are a great help during the Attack period. I recommend that you always have a few hard-boiled eggs to hand in the fridge.

Boiled eggs
3 minutes for soft-boiled eggs
4 minutes for slightly firmer eggs
6–7 minutes for hard-boiled eggs

OEUFS BROUILLÉS (SCRAMBLED EGGS)

(2 servings)

4 eggs, beaten
1 tablespoon skimmed milk
Salt and black pepper

Put the milk in a small saucepan and season with salt and pepper. Pour the eggs over the milk, continuing to stir them while they cook. Scrambled eggs should be soft and moist and not overcooked. You may add a few prawns, some smoked salmon or lean pieces of ham.

Cruise diet variations: You can add vegetables – mushrooms, asparagus tips, tomatoes, etc.

OEUFS FARCIS AUX CREVETTES (STUFFED EGGS WITH SHRIMPS)

(makes 12 egg halves, a good starter)

6 hard-boiled eggs
450g (1lb) shrimps, rinsed, cleaned, cooked and finely chopped (reserve 6 shrimps, cut in half, to garnish)
1 tablespoon Mayonnaise (see page 167)

Slice each cooled hard-boiled egg into two equal halves and remove the yolks. Blend the yolks with the finely chopped shrimp. Add a little mayonnaise and fill the egg whites with the mixture. Garnish each egg half with the reserved shrimps.

ASPIC D'OEUF AU JAMBON (JELLIED EGGS AND HAM)

(4 servings)

4 x 4-minute soft-boiled eggs, peeled
4 slices extra-lean ham
1 x 7g (¼oz) packet unflavoured gelatine
125ml (4fl oz) cold water
225ml (8fl oz) boiling water
1 drop cognac
Salt and black pepper

First, make up some gelatine. Sprinkle gelatine flakes into the cold water and allow 1–2 minutes to soften. Add the hot water and stir until thoroughly dissolved. Add salt, pepper and one drop of brandy. Wrap each soft-boiled egg in half a slice of ham while it is still warm and place in a dish. Pour over the liquid gelatine and allow to cool.

SOUFFLÉ AU JAMBON
(HAM SOUFFLÉ)

(4 servings)

200g (7oz) extra-lean ham, cut into thin strips
200ml (7fl oz) skimmed milk
20g (¾oz) cornflour
4 eggs
400g (14oz) non-fat fromage frais or quark
1 pinch nutmeg
Salt and black pepper

Preheat the oven to 220°C/425°F/Gas 7.
Blend the cold milk with the cornflour. Separate the egg whites from the yolks. Beat together the yolks and fromage frais or quark and pour over the milk, stirring all the time until it thickens. Then add the ham, season and add the nutmeg. Beat the egg whites until very stiff and gently fold into the ham mixture. Adjust the seasoning and pour the mixture into a non-stick soufflé dish. Bake in the oven for 45 minutes.

FLAN (CUSTARD)

(6 servings)

5 eggs
1 fresh vanilla pod, split lengthwise
375ml (13fl oz) skimmed milk
1 tablespoon vanilla extract

1 teaspoon ground nutmeg
1 freshly grated nutmeg

Preheat the oven to 150°C/300°F/Gas 2.

Beat the eggs in a large bowl. Scrape out the inside of the vanilla pod and add this and the bean to the milk. Heat the milk without letting it boil. Remove the vanilla pod, and slowly pour the hot milk over the eggs, adding the vanilla extract and ground nutmeg. Pour the mixture into a soufflé dish, or into individual ramekins. Grate the nutmeg over each one. Place the soufflé dish or ramekins in a large baking dish, fill three-quarters of the way up with boiling water. Bake in this *bain-marie* for 30–35 minutes. Allow the custards to cool in the *bain-marie* for 2 hours before serving.

CAFÉ, CHOCOLATE OR VANILLA CRÈME

(4 servings)

3 eggs, separated
1/8 teaspoon cornflour
225ml (8fl oz) skimmed milk
Flavouring (choose one): 1 teaspoon instant coffee,
   1 teaspoon non-fat cocoa powder dissolved in
water or 1 vanilla pod, split lengthwise, insides
removed and mixed with a few drops of vanilla extract
Aspartame, to taste

First make the 'crème anglaise': in a bowl, mix the egg yolks with the cornflour and beat until you have a smooth mousse. Pour the milk into a saucepan and add the flavouring of your choice. Warm over a low heat. Remove from the heat. Add the warmed milk mixture to the egg yolks. Put back on a low heat and stir well until the mixture thickens. Turn off the heat as soon as the mixture sticks to the spatula. Aspartame may be added to sweeten. Pour into a large soufflé dish or individual ramekins. Allow to set in the refrigerator. Serve very cold. This can also be put into an ice-cream maker (follow the manufacturer's instructions).

ILE FLOTTANTE (FLOATING ISLAND)

(4 servings)

4 eggs, separated
500ml (18fl oz) skimmed milk
1 vanilla pod, split lengthwise
Aspartame, to taste

In a mixing bowl, beat the egg whites until they form soft but firm peaks (you can use a dash of cream of tartar to make this easier). In a saucepan bring the milk and a small vanilla pod to the boil. With a ladle carefully spoon out snowball-sized portions of the egg whites and drop them into the hot milk. They will swell up. After turning them over remove them with a slotted spoon and let them drain on a plate.

Beat the egg yolks and add the milk from the saucepan. Put this mixture over a low heat, stirring constantly. When it starts to thicken, quickly remove it from the heat or it will curdle. Sweeten with aspartame powder. Let it cool. Put the mixture in a glass bowl then place the egg-white snowballs delicately on the surface. Serve chilled.

Vegetable-only Recipes for the Cruise Diet

CHOU-FLEUR (CAULIFLOWER)
(4 servings)

1 fresh cauliflower, washed thoroughly
Sauce Blanche (see page 168)
2 hard-boiled eggs, to serve

Cut the cauliflower into large pieces and cook in a large pan with salted water. When cooked, drain carefully. Pour the white sauce over the cauliflower. Serve with hard-boiled eggs cut in half.

SOUFFLÉ DE CHOU-FLEUR
(CAULIFLOWER SOUFFLÉ)

(main course for 2 or a side dish for 4)

1 fresh cauliflower, washed thoroughly
Sauce Blanche (see page 168)
2 eggs, separated

Preheat the oven to 200°C/400°F/Gas 6.
Cut the cauliflower into large pieces and cook in salted water until soft. Drain well. Make the white sauce (see page 168), but add two extra egg yolks. Beat the egg whites into a foam (do not overbeat) and fold them slowly into the white sauce. Put the cauliflower in a soufflé dish, pour over the sauce and bake for 20 minutes.

FRICASSÉE DE CHAMPIGNONS
(MUSHROOM FRICASSEE)

(side dish for 4)

450g (1lb) fresh mushrooms (chanterelle, oyster, portabella, etc.)
140g (5oz) chopped onion
1 low-fat chicken bouillon, dissolved in 50ml (2fl oz) hot water
1 garlic clove, diced
15g (½oz) parsley, chopped
Salt and black pepper

In a non-stick frying pan sauté the onion in the bouillon water mixture until almost caramelized. Remove the stems and cut the mushrooms into thick slices. Add the mushrooms to the pan and cook slowly over a low heat, uncovered, so that the liquid slowly evaporates and the mushrooms become plump and soft. Add garlic, parsley, salt and pepper. Serve hot with meat or poultry.

CHAMPIGNONS FARCIS (STUFFED MUSHROOMS)

(makes 20 hors d'oeuvres)

20 large mushrooms, washed
2 garlic cloves, chopped
30g (1oz) parsley, chopped
A few teaspoons of skimmed milk
A few drops of vegetable oil
Salt and black pepper

Preheat the oven to 200°C/400°F/Gas 6.

Use the largest mushrooms you can find. Wash and remove the stalks. Chop the stalks and add the garlic, parsley, salt, pepper and skimmed milk. Cook the stuffing mixture in a non-stick frying pan. Meanwhile, bake the mushroom caps stem side down for 10 minutes. Fill the hollow mushroom caps with the cooked stuffing and then bake in the oven for about 20 minutes or until done. When cooked drizzle a drop or two of vegetable oil over each stuffed mushroom.

EPINARDS SAUCE BLANCHE
(SPINACH WITH WHITE SAUCE)

(side dish for 6)

450g (1lb) fresh spinach leaves, rinsed
1 litre (1¾ pints) lightly salted water
Sauce Blanche (see page 168)

Preheat the oven to 180°C/350°F/Gas 4.
Wash the spinach leaves and cook them in boiling salted water for 10–15 minutes. Drain completely, and crush the leaves with a slotted spoon. Add the white sauce and bake in the oven for 40 minutes. Serve with hard-boiled eggs cut into halves or with meat or poultry.

Fennel

Fennel is a marvellous vegetable with a delicate taste of liquorice. It has great nutritional value and is also extremely rich in antioxidants. You can eat it raw – it makes a lovely salad – cut into diagonal slices and served with diet vinaigrette. It can also be cooked, if boiled very slowly but thoroughly, to soften its resistant fibres. It tastes very good with a dash of lemon juice and parsley. Serve at room temperature or slightly warm.

French beans

The diet-food award-winner, this vegetable has the fewest calories, but is rich in pectin, which makes us feel full. Even so, dieters often overlook French beans because when steamed they lose their colour and do not look so appetizing. Do not forget to use them as a salad ingredient, with a vinaigrette, or chopped onion and parsley. You can mix them with other more colourful vegetables such as tomatoes or raw peppers. Serve them in a white sauce or on their own to accompany meat or poultry.

TOMATES FAÇON MOZZARELLA BASILIC (STUFFED TOMATOES)

(2 main servings, or starter for 4)

225g (8oz) non-fat cottage cheese
2 large beef tomatoes, halved
Fresh basil leaves
Vinaigrette (see page 166)
Salt and black pepper

Strain off the liquid from the cottage cheese, then leave at room temperature for a few hours so that it attains a more solid consistency, like that of Italian mozzarella or Greek feta cheese. Halve the tomatoes, scoop out the seeds and fill with the cottage cheese. Top each one with a basil leaf, salt, pepper and vinaigrette.

CUCUMBERS – SERVED HOT OR COLD

(side dish for 4, starter for 2)

To prepare hot:
2 cucumbers
50ml (2fl oz) vinegar
Sauce Blanche (see page 168)
Salt

Wash, peel and slice the cucumbers. Cook on a high heat for 10 minutes in water mixed with the vinegar. Add a little salt. Drain well, and serve with the white sauce.

To serve cold in a salad:
2 cucumbers
Vinaigrette (see page 166)
1 small onion, sliced

Remove all the seeds from the cucumbers, then slice them and leave to drain in a colander for 1 hour. Serve with the vinaigrette and a few sliced onions.

ENDIVES EN SALADE
(CHICORY SALAD WITH SPECIAL DRESSING)

(2 servings)

Chicory is a low-calorie vegetable, great for anyone on a diet who doesn't have time to cook at lunchtime as it is so easy to use and carry around. Chicory has a delicate, slightly bitter taste, and is deliciously fresh and crunchy.

This is why it is possible to prepare a special dressing for use only with chicory, a sauce that breaks our normally stringent rules and permits on this one occasion a new food that in other circumstances would be considered dangerous for a diet – Roquefort cheese. Use the part of the cheese that is the darkest and the strongest in its grey-blue colour. To reassure you about this minor transgression: one small teaspoon of Roquefort contains no more fat than one black olive.

175g (6oz) non-fat yoghurt
1 teaspoon white wine vinegar
1 teaspoon Roquefort cheese (the dark blue part)
4 chicory heads, washed and sliced

Mix together the yoghurt, vinegar and cheese until smooth. Pour the sauce on the chicory and serve.

ENDIVES BRAISES (BRAISED CHICORY)

(side dish for 4)

4 chicory heads, trimmed and cut in half
1 small onion, sliced
1 low-fat beef bouillon cube, dissolved in
*   50ml (2fl oz) water*

Wash and steam the chicory. In a non-stick frying pan, sauté a few onion slices with the bouillon cube and water. Add the drained chicory and simmer until golden brown. Serve warm with the pan juices. It goes well with white meat, such as veal or turkey.

ENDIVES GRATINÉES (CHICORY GRATIN)
(side dish for 4)

450g (1lb) chicory, trimmed
Sauce Blanche (see page 168)
1 egg, beaten
Salt

Preheat the oven to 190°C/375°F/Gas 5.
Wash and steam the chicory. Add salt and drain. Place the chicory in a baking dish with the white sauce. Beat an egg and pour it over the bed of chicory. Bake in the oven for 25 minutes until the top is golden brown.

ASPERGES SAUCE MOUSSELINE (ASPARAGUS WITH MOUSSELINE SAUCE)
(side dish for 4)

1 bundle fresh asparagus
1 egg white
Mayonnaise (see page 167)
A dash of raspberry vinegar

Prepare the fresh asparagus by scraping off the stringy fibres at the ends. Place in a saucepan with water and steam for 20–25 minutes. Beat the egg white into peaks and mix it into the mayonnaise until completely smooth. Add a dash of raspberry vinegar, which will make the sauce slightly more liquid. Serve the asparagus warm, garnished with the mousseline sauce.

AUBERGINES À L'INDIENNE (INDIAN-STYLE AUBERGINES)

(2 servings)

200g (7oz) aubergines, thinly sliced
50g (1¾oz) tomatoes, finely chopped
1 tablespoon herbes de Provence (mixed herbs)
1 pinch curry powder
1 pinch paprika
1 handful coriander
50g (1¾oz) red pepper, thinly sliced
Salt and black pepper

Simmer the tomatoes in a non-stick pan over a gentle heat until cooked. Season with salt and pepper, and add the herbs and spices. Blanch the aubergines and red pepper for few minutes then leave to cool. Place a layer of cooked aubergines then a layer of peppers in an ovenproof dish. Pour the tomato sauce over the top. Bake in the oven for 10 minutes at 220°C/425°F/ Gas 7.

SOUPE MIRACULEUSE (MIRACLE SOUP)

(8–10 servings)

This is a soup that goes beyond the boundaries of our normal instructions and is based on recent research that has proved the long-term effectiveness of lumpy vegetable soup.

4 garlic cloves
6 large onions
1 or 2 tins peeled tomatoes
1 large cabbage head
6 carrots
2 green peppers
1 bunch celery
3 litres (5¼ pints) water
3 low-fat beef bouillon cubes
3 low-fat chicken bouillon cubes.

Peel and cut the vegetables into equal-size pieces. Put them in a soup pot with the stock cube and cover with water. Let them boil for 10 minutes, then reduce the heat and continue cooking until the vegetables are tender.

This soup is extremely filling and the chunky pieces of vegetable are the reason for its weight-loss properties. The liquid and the solid elements go through the digestive tract at varying speeds. The solid pieces remain in the stomach until they are totally digested; they fill you up and produce a physical feeling of being full. The liquid goes through the stomach more quickly and arrives in the small intestine, where its nutritional ingredients stimulate the intestinal walls and generate a feeling of satisfaction. The combination of feeling full in the stomach and the metabolic feeling of satisfaction in the small intestine works to reduce appetite, quickly, noticeably and on a long-term basis.

This soup is highly recommended for those people who arrive home starving after a long day at work because they only ate a tiny lunch or skipped lunch altogether. Such people can't resist snacking on something right away, which is often as rich in fats as it is enjoyable, thereby spoiling their efforts to lose weight. One bowl of this soup, served hot, and you will find that these cravings disappear and you are able comfortably to wait for your dinner to arrive.

SOUPE AU POTIRON (PUMPKIN SOUP)

(10–12 servings)

¼ pumpkin, peeled and cut into large pieces
1 large onion
1 apple, peeled and cored
1 low-fat chicken bouillon cube
1 tablespoon curry powder
115g (4oz) non-fat fromage frais or quark
Salt and black pepper

Put the pumpkin, onion, apple and bouillon cube in a pressure cooker, cover with water and cook for 20–30 minutes. After cooking, purée the soup in a blender but do not make it too smooth, so that you can still taste some bits of pumpkin melt in your mouth. Add salt, pepper, curry powder and mix in the non-fat fromage frais or quark.

SOUPE ONCTUEUSE AUX COURGETTES (THICK COURGETTE SOUP)

(6–8 servings)

4 large courgettes, washed and peeled
1 large onion
1 carrot, wash and peeled
1 turnip, washed
1 low-fat beef bouillon cube

Wash, peel and cut the vegetables into large pieces. Put in a tall pan with the low-fat beef bouillon cube and cover with water. Cook for 20–30 minutes. Purée using a blender to obtain a thick, smooth soup. Serve hot.

Vegetable + Protein Recipes for the Cruise Phase

SALADE DES ROIS DE LA MER (KINGS OF THE SEA SALAD)

(4 servings)

1 lettuce head, cut into pieces
115g (4oz) each of smoked salmon, cooked shrimp,
  crab, crab sticks (surimi), octopus, smoked
  haddock, salmon roe and lumpfish roe
Vinaigrette (see page 166)
Salt and black pepper

Put the lettuce in a large salad bowl and add the smoked salmon cut in strips, a handful of shrimps, crab pieces, two chopped crab sticks, pieces of octopus and strips of smoked haddock. Season with salt and pepper, and serve with our vinaigrette, decorated with a mixture of salmon roe and lumpfish roe.

SALADE AU POULET SAUCE YAOURT AUX HERBES (CHICKEN AND YOGHURT HERB SAUCE SALAD)

(2 servings)

300g (10½oz) button mushrooms
1 bunch radishes

4 slices cooked chicken breast
4 large gherkins, cut into thick slices
1 small pot non-fat yoghurt
1 garlic clove, chopped
1 teaspoon mustard
A few sprigs of parsley, finely chopped
A few chives, finely chopped
Salt and black pepper

Wash the mushrooms and radishes and cut into small cubes. Cut the chicken into strips and add the gherkins. Make up the sauce by mixing the yoghurt with the garlic, mustard, parsley and chives, salt and pepper. Pour into a dish, mix all the ingredients together and keep in a cool place until served.

SALADE COMPOSÉE (MIXED SALAD)
(4 servings)

1 lettuce head, cut into pieces
2 tomatoes, sliced
1 hard-boiled egg, cut into quarters
115g (4oz) chopped white chicken meat
2 lean slices ham (trimmed), chopped
Vinaigrette (see page 166)

Mix the lettuce together with the tomatoes, hard-boiled egg, chicken and ham. Serve with vinaigrette.

THON AUX TROIS POIVRONS (THREE PEPPER TUNA)

(2 servings)

700g (1lb 9oz) tuna steak
1 red pepper
1 green pepper
1 yellow pepper
Juice of 1–2 lemons
2 garlic cloves, crushed
Salt and white pepper

Wash, de-seed and halve the peppers. Put them under the grill for 5 minutes, then to make peeling them easier place in a plastic bag for 10 minutes. Next cut them into strips and gently fry for a few minutes over a moderate heat in a non-stick frying pan that has been lightly oiled (add some oil then wipe with kitchen paper) with a little water in the bottom. Season the tuna and steam for 20 minutes. Mix together the lemon juice, garlic and peppers. When the tuna is cooked, allow to cool then marinate it with the peppers in a cool place for 2–3 hours, turning the tuna regularly. Serve cold.

BROCHETTE DE BOEUF TURGLOFF
(TURGLOFF BEEF KEBAB)

(2 servings)

600g (1lb 5oz) lean beef
500g (1lb 2oz) tomatoes, peeled and de-seeded
1 garlic clove, crushed
200g (7oz) peppers
200g (7oz) onions
Juice of 1 lemon
Celery salt
Tarragon salt
Salt and black pepper
Fresh parsley, to garnish

Crush the tomatoes and simmer with the garlic in a frying pan over a gentle heat. Season. Cut the meat, peppers and onions into chunks. Put them on to kebab sticks and grill for about 10 minutes either on the barbecue or under the grill. When you are ready to serve, remove the ingredients from the sticks, sprinkle with lemon juice and add some celery and tarragon salt. Pour a little of the tomato sauce on to each plate. Adjust the seasoning and garnish with parsley.

VEAU AUX ENDIVES (VEAL WITH CHICORY)

(4 servings)

450g (1lb) lean veal escalopes or 4 veal chops,
    trimmed of fat
1 medium onion, sliced
1 low-fat chicken bouillon cube, dissolved in
    50ml (2fl oz) water
4 chicory heads, washed and steamed
Salt and black pepper

Place a layer of sliced onions, with the chicken bouillon and water, in a non-stick frying pan. Cook over a low heat until the onions are golden in colour. Place the veal escalopes or veal chops on top of the bed of onions and cook slowly, until the veal is golden brown. Add the cooked chicory leaves, season and simmer over a low heat for 1 hour. Serve hot. Put any leftovers in the refrigerator to be eaten cold with Dijon mustard or reheated for another meal.

POULET AUX CHAMPIGNONS (CHICKEN WITH MUSHROOMS)

(4 servings)

4 small boneless chicken breasts
1 medium onion, sliced
175g (6oz) sliced mushrooms

1 low-fat chicken bouillon cube, dissolved in
   50ml (2fl oz) water
4 chicory heads, washed and steamed
Salt and black pepper

Place a layer of sliced onions and mushrooms, with the chicken bouillon and water, in a non-stick frying pan. Cook over a low heat until the onions are golden in colour. Place the chicken breasts on top of the bed of onions and mushrooms, and cook slowly. Add the cooked chicory leaves, season and simmer over a low heat for 1 hour. Serve hot. Put any leftovers in the refrigerator to be eaten cold with Dijon mustard or reheated for another meal.

POULET MARENGO (CHICKEN MARENGO)

(4 servings)

4 boneless chicken breasts, cut into pieces
1 medium onion, sliced
1 low-fat chicken bouillon cube, dissolved in 50ml (2fl oz) water
2 tomatoes, cut into pieces
¼ teaspoon thyme
125ml (4fl oz) dry white wine
30g (1oz) mushrooms, washed and sliced
Salt and black pepper

In a non-stick frying pan, prepare a bed of sliced onions with the bouillon cube dissolved in a little water. Simmer until golden in colour. Add the tomatoes and thyme, and season. Place the chicken pieces on this soft onion and tomato layer. Add the wine, cover and cook over a low heat for 1 hour. Add the mushrooms 30 minutes into the cooking. To finish, reduce the excess liquid by rapidly boiling the pan juices uncovered for a few seconds.

RABBIT MEDALLIONS WITH MUSHROOMS

(4 servings)

450g (1lb) rabbit medallions
1 medium onion, chopped
175g (6oz) mushrooms, sliced
1 low-fat beef bouillon cube, dissolved in 50ml (2fl oz) water
¼ teaspoon dried thyme
¼ teaspoon dried rosemary
125ml (4fl oz) dry white wine
Black pepper

Pound the rabbit medallions between two sheets of plastic wrap until 1cm (½in) thick. In a non-stick frying pan, prepare a bed of onions and mushrooms in a little water with the bouillon cube and herbs. Leave over a low heat until the mushrooms turn a golden colour. Place the rabbit medallions on the bottom of the pan, and sauté until the meat is brown. Add the wine, cover and cook slowly for 20 minutes. When the mushrooms have lost all their moisture, cook on a high heat for several seconds to thicken the sauce. Serve with freshly ground black pepper.

OEUFS AUX CHAMPIGNONS (EGG FRITTATA)

(4 servings)

225g (8oz) fresh mushrooms, washed and sliced
140g (5oz) chopped onion
5 large eggs, beaten

Preheat the oven to 180°C/350°F/Gas 4.
Sauté the mushrooms and onions in a non-stick frying pan. Combine with the eggs in a soufflé dish and bake, covered with foil, for 45 minutes.

SANDWICH DUKAN AU POULET ET À L'OMELETTE AUX HERBES (DUKAN CHICKEN AND HERB OMELETTE SANDWICH)

(1 serving)

2 tablespoons oat bran
1 tablespoon wheat bran
1 teaspoon baking powder
2 tablespoons non-fat fromage frais or quark plus
    extra for spreading
2 eggs plus 1 egg white

1 tablespoon chopped parsley
Herbs of your choice (e.g. basil, herbes de Provence/
*   mixed herbs, shallots)*
Chopped cooked chicken breast

In a rectangular bowl, thoroughly mix the brans, baking powder, fromage frais or quark and 1 egg. Add the chopped parsley and heat in the microwave (800W) for 4 minutes. Turn out and allow to cool a little before cutting the 'bread' into 2 slices and toasting very lightly so that it does not go dry. Make an omelette with the remaining egg, the egg white, and the herbs. Fold over the four edges to make a rectangle. Spread each slice of bread with fromage frais or quark. Make up the sandwich by putting the chopped chicken on the bottom slice then placing the omelette on top and covering with the top slice of bread.

One Week of Menus for the Pure Protein Attack Phase

BREAKFAST – For Every Day of the Week

Coffee or tea with aspartame
+ choice of: 1 or 2 small non-fat yoghurts or 225g (8oz) non-fat cottage cheese
+ choice of: 1 slice turkey, chicken or low-fat ham; or 1 egg; or 1 egg custard; or 1 Dukan oat bran galette (see page 76).

AT 10 or 11 a.m. (if hungry)

1 small non-fat yoghurt or 115g (4oz) non-fat cottage cheese

AT 4 p.m. (if necessary)

1 non-fat yoghurt or 1 slice of turkey or both

Suggestion: make enough food for dinner, so you can have it for lunch the next day – or within the next two days.

MONDAY

Lunch	Dinner
Hard-boiled egg with Dukan mayonnaise	Shrimps Sautéed in Herbs
Pepper Steak	Tandoori Chicken Escalopes
2 non-fat yoghurts or 225g (8oz) fromage frais/quark	Custard or 1 non-fat yoghurt

Lunch
Hard-boiled egg with
    Dukan mayonnaise
Pepper Steak
2 non-fat yoghurts or 225g
    (8oz) fromage frais/quark

Dinner
Shrimps Sautéed in Herbs
Tandoori Chicken Escalopes
Custard or 1 non-fat yoghurt

TUESDAY

Lunch
Marinated Raw Salmon
Luc Lac Beef
2 non-fat yoghurts

Dinner
Stuffed Crab
Chicken with Mustard
Custard or 1 non-fat yoghurt

WEDNESDAY

Lunch
Crab sticks
Chicken leg
Custard or 1 Dukan oat
    bran galette

Dinner
Jellied Eggs and Ham
White Fish with White Sauce
Floating Island or 225g (8oz)
    fromage frais/quark

THURSDAY

Lunch
1 slice smoked salmon
Sautéed Veal Chops

Dinner
Scampi with Mayonnaise
Ham Soufflé

Chocolate Crème or
   225g (8oz) fromage
   frais/quark

Custard or 1 non-
   fat yoghurt

FRIDAY

Lunch
4 slices wind-dried beef
Grilled swordfish
2 non-fat yoghurts or
   225g (8oz) fromage
   frais/quark

Dinner
Jellied Eggs and Ham
Indian chicken
Floating Island or
   2 non-fat yoghurts

SATURDAY

Lunch
Scrambled Eggs
Poached Salmon Fillets
Custard or 1 Dukan oat
   bran galette

Dinner
Moules Marinières
Lemon Chicken
Floating Island or
225g (8oz) fromage frais/
   quark

SUNDAY

Lunch
Stuffed Eggs with Shrimps
Meat Loaf
Café Crème or Custard

Dinner
Salmon Tartar
Boiled Beef
Floating Island or 225g
   (8oz) fromage frais/quark

One Week of Menus for Pure Proteins Followed by Pure Proteins + Vegetables

The breakfasts, mid-morning and afternoon snacks for the entire week are the same as the Attack-only phase.

MONDAY

Lunch	*Dinner*
Smoked salmon	Stuffed Eggs with Shrimps
Baked Salmon	Chicken Soufflé
Custard or 1 Dukan oat bran galette	Café Crème or 225g (8oz) fromage frais/quark

TUESDAY

Lunch	*Dinner*
Stuffed Mushrooms	Pumpkin Soup
Three Pepper Tuna	Turgloff Beef Kebab
2 non-fat yoghurts or 225g (8oz) fromage frais/quark	Custard or 1 non-fat yoghurt

WEDNESDAY

Lunch	*Dinner*
Jellied Eggs and Ham	Shrimps Sautéed in Herbs
Baked Salmon	Chicken with Mustard
Custard or 1 Dukan oat bran galette	Floating Island or 225g (8oz) fromage frais/quark

THURSDAY

Lunch
Stuffed Tomatoes
Dukan Chicken and Herb
   Omelette Sandwich
Café Crème or 225g (8oz)
   fromage frais/quark

Dinner
Thick Courgette Soup
Baked Salmon Parcel
Custard or 1 non-fat
   yoghurt

FRIDAY

Lunch
Hard-boiled egg with
   mayonnaise
Boiled Beef
2 non-fat yoghurts or 225g
   (8oz) fromage frais/quark

Dinner
Meat Loaf
Grilled Sea Bream
Floating Island or Custard

SATURDAY

Lunch
Chicory Salad with
   Special Dressing
Cauliflower Soufflé
   and grilled steak
Custard or 1 Dukan oat
   bran galette

Dinner
Indian-style Aubergines
Chicken Marengo
Vanilla Crème or 225g (8oz)
   fromage frais/quark

SUNDAY

Lunch

Mixed Salad with tuna
Veal with Chicory
Floating Island

Dinner

Asparagus with Mousseline
   Sauce
Chicken and Yoghurt Herb
   Sauce Salad
Chocolate Crème or Custard

MAJOR OBESITY

SOME EXCEPTIONAL
EXTRA MEASURES

The programme that I have shown you here is for everyone whose quality of life is impaired by weight problems they find hard to control, which covers a great variety of individuals who are all different yet can be divided into three categories according to the amount of weight involved.

From a Few Extra Pounds to Major Obesity

Putting on extra pounds occasionally

This category includes anyone who does not have a predisposition to being overweight, whose weight has always been normal and stable, but who has started to put on extra pounds due to a specific, identifiable reason – that is, suddenly stopping taking exercise.

This is what happens after women give birth, usually with their first child, when understandably caught up in the excitement and unable to take normal exercise they put on weight. This is even more common if the birth has been difficult, requiring prolonged bed rest, or if the mother has had IVF or other fertility treatment.

It can also happen to anyone who is temporarily immobilized by an accident and eats out of sheer boredom. This category also includes people receiving cortisone treatment for asthma or rheumatism.

Predisposition to obesity

These are men and women who are predisposed to put on weight. Whether this is 'inherited', or because of overfeeding in early childhood leading to bad eating habits, the results are the same. These people have a tendency to put on pounds easily and extract an excessive amount of calories from what they eat.

In roughly 90 per cent of cases, this predisposition is moderate and the excessive calorie extraction is manageable.

In this category, some individuals, who have strong willpower and motivation, manage to watch what they eat, lead an active lifestyle and can stop the pounds piling on or at least keep them under control. My programme offers such men and women real security, freeing them forever from their legitimate anxiety about their weight. But where the Dukan Diet can really help them is to get through those unavoidable critical periods in life when simple willpower is just not enough.

Others, who suffer from the same predisposition to put on weight but who are sedentary or have no self-control when eating, experience a slow but inevitable increase in weight. For them the Dukan Diet is ideal; they extract a high level of calories from their food but the combination of protein Thursdays and regular consumption of oat bran completely neutralizes this problem. Their lack of willpower or organized eating patterns is balanced by this one semi-heroic day, when for a small sacrifice they can put themselves through a sort of weekly redemption.

Major obesity

Major obesity is a predisposition that often runs in the family, leading to such huge weight gain that the body is deformed – very common in the USA but still rare in Europe.

With these seriously obese people, the energy they absorb from what they eat is so great that everyone, doctors included, are stupefied. All nutritionists have some such patients who seem to live off thin air, defying the most elementary laws of physics.

I have known patients who have weighed themselves before going to bed and who immediately on waking up and even before urinating had found a way of putting on a little weight. These cases exist and perplex doctors, but fortunately they are the rare exceptions.

Most often, individuals with a strong predisposition to gain weight are clearly obese. It is here that we encounter people who have already tried most diets, almost always losing weight which they then put straight back on again. For them, the fourth phase of the programme is a good basis for stabilization but it is unlikely to be sufficient in the most difficult cases. So for this reason, in this chapter dedicated to them, I suggest a series of extra measures to shore up their stabilization.

But, in line with my original philosophy, these measures are not based on restricting what you eat. Everything that I have recommended from the beginning in this book remains valid, even for those with a special talent for extracting calories. After a successful diet, eating during stabilization must be spontaneous six days out of seven.

The three measures that follow are of course intended particularly for anyone with an extreme tendency to obesity resulting in massive, deforming and uncontrollable weight gain. But what is good for them may also help those people who, although not obese, already have a 'weight history' and are looking for effective control.

Vital Information You Need to Know Beforehand

Nowadays we know that we are born with a genetically determined supply of adipocytes, those infamous yellow cells that make and store fat. Normally the number of these cells is fixed and does not vary. It is interesting to know that, although this number is fixed, it does vary for individuals and those with more of them have a greater capacity to put on weight.

Genetically women have more adipocytes than men as fat plays a more important role in expressing a woman's femininity as well as in reproduction and motherhood. A woman with less than ten per cent of fat reserves stops ovulating to prevent her from starting a pregnancy she will not have the energy to sustain to term.

Once the number of these adipocytes has been determined at birth it then remains relatively constant –

except for certain key moments that I would like to draw your attention to.

When a woman – or a man – who eats badly or too much puts on weight, their adipocytes put on weight too. As the person continues to put on weight, their adipocytes continue to gorge themselves on fat, gradually becoming distended. If the weight gain continues, the adipocytes hypertrophy, or enlarge, and reach the limit of their elasticity. At this critical moment, any additional weight gain triggers a new and exceptional event, completely changing the future and prognosis for weight problems. No longer able to contain any more fat the adipocyte cell DIVIDES into two daughter adipocyte cells. This simple division suddenly doubles the body's capacity to make and store fat.

From this moment on, the tendency to put on weight increases; quite simply it becomes easier to put it on and more difficult to take it off. This is because, if you are trying to lose weight, you can always reduce the size of the adipocytes but the two daughter cells will never again become a single mother cell.

Nutritionists know this but the general public does not and it is vital that they do, especially those whose weight gain is moderate. It is important to stop them from going past this point of no return when the struggle becomes much harder in a more challenging environment. When the adipocytes divide, what was excess weight through behaviour becomes metabolic excess weight and nothing will ever be as simple as it was before.

I am not writing this to make anyone who is obese feel worried or guilty, although losing weight for them is more difficult and takes longer than before. I can reassure them that, while realizing their limits, my method does give them the means to deal with their resistance.

Having said this, for those who are in danger and to whom this applies, it is important to pinpoint simply and concretely the moment in their weight history when there is this risk of cell division – so that they do not reach it.

Having worked with tens of thousands of patients throughout my career as a nutritionist, and using a precise parameter – the time when obvious and sudden resistance to dieting and weight loss appeared – I was able to work out statistics that enabled me to pinpoint this moment as being after BMI 28 has been reached and going towards BMI 29.

Calculating your BMI

You need to know what your BMI is and how to calculate it. You calculate your BMI, or Body Mass Index, by dividing your weight by your height squared. So, for example, if you weigh 11 stone (70kg) and are 5ft 3in (1.6m) the calculation is – using metric which is easier – 1.6 x 1.6 = 2.56; 70 ÷ 2.56 = 27.34. (There are also many websites that will calculate your BMI for you.)

This BMI has not yet reached 28 but it is not far off – just a few more pounds will take it to 28 and beyond. The main thing is to do all you can to avoid ever reaching this danger point.

If you do not already know your BMI, work it out as it could not be easier. Then watch it closely and when you get near to BMI 27 be careful and do not allow yourself to go any further as your adipocytes are very full. And if you do reach 28, do something: your adipocytes are at saturation point and are likely to divide at any moment, making managing and controlling your weight more complicated.

So now you know and I ask you to tell your friends and children about it. I hope that this book will help spread this vital piece of information.

Exceptional Measure No. 1: Using the Cold to Control Weight

Throughout the programme that I have just described to you, we tackled your weight problem with dieting and oat bran, which creates calorie loss in the intestines. Then we used exercise, especially the quintessential human activity of walking, to burn off calories. Still with the same objective of increasing the body's calorie expenditure, here is an unusual way of burning calories, a very original and little known method to which I attach much importance: making the body use up calories by keeping itself warm.

If we imagine a 13 stone man, 5ft 9in tall, with a semi-active profession, during his normal routine he eats and uses up on average about 2,400 calories a day.

Let's try and pinpoint exactly how and where he uses these calories:

- 300 calories per day ensure that vital organs and functions work: the heart, brain, liver, kidneys, etc. Very little energy is used for all this, showing how well our organs are adapted to survive; so we cannot get our bodies to increase energy consumption here.

- 700 calories are needed for motor activity and movement. Plainly we have the means of increasing this activity. For a long time I made the same mistake as everyone else and only *recommended* more exercise, which allowed me – along with all the others giving advice – to ease my conscience, but this did no good. As time went by, and faced with my daily battle against weight problems, I realized how vitally important exercise is for losing weight and, even more so, for stabilizing in the long term.

  I have therefore made walking one of the sacred tenets of my method. Now, I no longer 'recommend' walking I 'prescribe' it, with the same solemnity and total conviction as I would for any medicine. This walking, which I set apart from all other physical effort, is fundamentally human, written into our genes.

- 1,400 calories, the main amount, covers our metabolic requirements, and over half is used to keep our central body temperature at around 37°C/98.6°F, essential for our survival. This is then the area where we can and will increase energy consumption.

To do this we just have to accept the idea that the cold can become a friend and ally of the obese. Long gone are the days when humans warmed themselves by open fires. We have long since conquered the cold, sparing our bodies the task of keeping us warm by employing a whole range of external protection (central heating, clothes) which nowadays we too often take to extremes. Our bodies being no longer adapted to cope with the cold, when forced to do so they burn up huge amounts of calories just to maintain our vital internal temperature. To help stabilize your weight, we can make use of this inability to cope with the cold which results in burning up energy. Studies show that the average Westerner is overprotected against the cold, and the obese, with their layer of fat, even more so.

The technique I suggest here aims to counter your ability to store calories by increasing what you use to keep yourself warm, and consists of a series of simple measures that have nothing to do with food restriction, but which are highly effective and will teach you how to use the cold to help maintain your weight stabilization. First and foremost, you need to know that so as not to die the human body has to maintain its temperature above 35°C/95°F. This is not a recommendation but rather an absolute, vital top priority.

Eat cold food as often as possible

When you put very hot food in your mouth, you absorb its calories. Without realizing it you also absorb the heat in the food and this heat provides extra calories that help maintain your body's temperature at 37°C/98.6°F.

Therefore, a hot steak is higher in calories than a cold steak because as soon as you start eating the hot meat, your body stops burning its own calories and uses the heat in the food.

On the other hand, when you eat cold food your body has to heat it up to body temperature before it can be absorbed into your bloodstream. This operation not only burns lots of calories, but also has the added advantage of slowing down digestion and assimilation, thereby delaying the return of your appetite.

Obviously, I am not advising you to eat cold food all the time, but whenever you have the choice between a hot or cold dish, choose the cold one.

Enjoy cold drinks

Eating cold food is not always pleasurable. However, having a cold drink is a simple habit to adopt and is already popular with a lot of people.

For any obese person, whose weight refuses to shift, this next measure is often agreeable and can prove very effective. When you take 2 litres of water from your fridge its temperature is 4°C/39.2°F. After you have drunk and assimilated it, you will then eliminate it in your urine at 37°C/98.6°F. To bring the temperature of this water up from 4°C/39.2°F to 37°C/98.6°F your body has to burn 60 calories. Once this becomes a habit, you can burn 22,000 calories a year, equivalent to almost six pounds and a godsend for anyone who finds stabilization difficult.

Conversely, a cup of very hot tea, even if you are careful to use artificial sweetener so that it is calorie-free, does nevertheless give you a dose of heat, which adds a few crafty calories that few people know about.

Suck on ice cubes

Research shows that ice works even better, if kept well below freezing (-10°C/14°F). Using this principle, I suggest that my patients make ice cubes sweetened with aspartame, vanilla or mint, and that they suck five or six a day – especially during hot weather, as this uses up 60 calories without any effort.

Slim in the shower

Try this simple experiment: take a shower holding a plastic thermometer (a glass one might slip out and break). Let the water run until the thermometer reads 25°C/77°F. What could you compare this temperature to? A pleasant dip in the sea in the summer!

If you stay under the shower for two minutes your body has to expend almost 100 calories just to prevent your body temperature from going down, the same amount you would use to walk about two miles.

This refreshing shower is most effective when the water is applied to the areas of the body where the blood circulating is the warmest: the armpits, groin, neck and chest, where the large warm arteries are nearest to the skin's surface, so most heat will be lost. Avoid getting your hair wet or showering your back in this temperature as it serves no purpose and can be unpleasant. If you are one of those people who are just too sensitive to the cold, you can still lose a few calories by showering those parts of your body that can handle cold temperatures: your thighs, legs and feet.

Avoid overheated environments

The obese person should realize that in winter an indoor temperature of 25°C/77°F encourages their tendency to put on weight. For anyone wanting to lose weight, lowering the temperature by 3°C/37.4°F can make their body burn an extra 100 calories a day, the equivalent of running for 20 minutes.

Do not wrap up so much

This idea stems from the preceding one, but it is possible to combine them. When the cold weather arrives, more often out of habit than necessity you get out all your sweaters and warm underwear. At night, many people put on extra blankets, less out of a real need for warmth than for the pleasure of feeling snug. Make a choice and get rid of at least one of these three protective layers: warm underwear, sweaters or extra bedcovers. You will burn up 100 calories every day by simply doing this.

If you tend towards obesity you should also be aware that wearing tight or clinging clothes is not recommended. We sweat a little when dressed; this is to refresh the body and to lower body temperature and should be encouraged by wearing clothes as loosely as possible.

Conclusion

By adding up all these ways of burning up energy we can understand the importance of using the cold to help stabilize difficult weights.

Drinking two litres of water at 10°C/50°F forces your body, to stop it cooling down, to burn	60 calories
Sucking six flavoured ice cubes	60 calories
A two-minute shower at 25°C/77°F	100 calories
Lowering the room temperature by 3°C/37.4°F	100 calories
Going without thermal underwear, a sweater or extra blanket	100 calories
Total	**420 calories**

The above list shows clearly how effective these measures are.

Any reader who doubts the reality of this must understand that I am talking about a physiological phenomenon and one that is highly logical. How can we possibly doubt that we use up calories to maintain our body temperature at 37°C/98.6°F and that this varies according to the ambient temperature and how cold it is? Everyone knows, from experience, just how much it costs to heat a badly insulated house. Our bodies work on the same principle, so we can make use of this and get the obese person to start using up some of those calories they like to hoard.

In conclusion, although cooling your body on its own is not enough to make an obese person lose weight, it can be very useful in a tricky Stabilization phase, when sometimes something very small can make all the difference and turn things round. Modest but regular calorie consumption to tackle the cold can be that little extra that guarantees success.

Finally, there is another reason that beats all the others by far and this is your own way to test the technique. Anyone who can see just how resistant their body is to losing weight and who follows my programme's permanent stabilization plan seriously and yet despite all their best efforts their hopes are not matched on their bathroom scales, should without a second thought try cooling down their body for a few weeks. After this short experiment, they will not need any more convincing.

For people who have a less extreme predisposition to obesity, this technique is not crucial. However, they can make use of it as and when, for example at risky times such as holidays, celebrations and parties, or they can select a cooling-down option they are comfortable with.

I would also like to add that confronting the cold can be a useful exercise for anyone who feels a weakness in certain areas of their psychological make-up, or who has a desire to strengthen their willpower in areas where they already feel strong. Facing up to cold temperatures can also help you face up to weaknesses in your eating habits.

To finish, I would say that heat and comfort soften you up; whereas the cold makes you dynamic, encourages muscular activity and strengthens the working of the thyroid. I have known many a depressed person begin to sing once they start taking a colder shower.

Exceptional Measure No. 2: Taking Useful Exercise

Most weight-loss theories recommend eating small quantities of food and increasing calorie expenditure by exercising at the same time. These recommendations seem logical and rational, but in practice they do not work. According to the American Association of Specialists in Obesity, 12 per cent of dieters actually do lose weight, but only two per cent succeed in keeping it off despite the enormous popularity of sport and exercise in America.

Do not practise sports during a period of intense weight loss

During the Dukan Diet's Attack phase and for as long as they are losing a lot of weight, I do not recommend that my obese patients undertake any sport or intense activity – although I do ask them TO WALK. There are three main reasons for this:

• The first is that the willpower required for dieting to be effective is challenging enough without asking for any extra concentrated effort that would risk jeopardizing the entire venture.

- The second reason is that an obese person who loses lots of weight feels more tired than usual, and needs rest and sleep to recover. Apart from walking, any extra physical activity is likely to increase tiredness and sap willpower.
- The third reason is that an obese person is by definition far too heavy for their body and forcing them to take uncustomary exercise to lose weight is quite simply dangerous.

An obese person is also quite understandably not enthusiastic about showing off their body by exercising in public.

Three minimum extra activities

Although intense exercise is excluded during weight loss, it does play a major role in the Stabilization phase once weight has been lost, to prevent the pounds from going back on and to firm up slack muscles and skin. Experience shows that getting an obese person to take regular exercise is no easy thing as their aversion to exercise and effort contributed to their obesity in the first place.

Nevertheless, I ask the seriously obese person who has managed to slim down but who finds stabilization difficult to add the following three simple rules to their basic programme. Everyone can use them, even those people who most hate taking exercise.

- Do not use lifts or escalators. I have already described this measure in the permanent Stabilization phase. There it was intended for anyone wanting to stabilize but here, for the obese person who has managed to reach their goal but realizes that they were not just dealing with a few extra pounds, this person who has achieved a great victory absolutely must include this measure now in their new lifestyle. They can take their time and stop halfway up to catch their breath; they can do what they like between the first and the last floors, but whatever they do they have to get there. I will remind you that any obese person who has lost weight is a much stronger individual than a person of normal weight because carrying around 20 to 25 stone all the time is permanent exercise, virtually a sport in itself. So once such a person has slimmed down, they still have the muscle mass and strength to make short work of the few floors that I recommend they walk up.
- Be on your feet as often as possible. Whenever you do not have to be sitting or lying down, consider standing up instead. To get the most out of this, distribute your weight evenly between each foot. Avoid leaning on one foot because then the weight is supported not by the muscles, which burn extra calories, but by the ligaments which do not.

  Do not overlook this seemingly insignificant advice. Standing up requires the static contraction of your body's largest muscles: the gluteus maximus, quadriceps and hamstrings. If every day you stand upright, balanced on both feet with your hips horizontal, this will burn up enough energy to make standing worthwhile.

- Walk with a purpose. This is a good opportunity to talk about walking again. You now know just how important it is in the battle against weight problems. You know that I prescribe a daily dose of 20 minutes for the Attack phase, 30 minutes in the Cruise phase with 60-minute boosters over four days to 'break through' a stagnation plateau. Then back to 25 minutes in Consolidation, finishing with a minimum of 20 minutes a day in the permanent Stabilization phase.

But for the victorious obese person these 20 minutes are not enough. As well as walking for its own sake, they must also add the hugely beneficial input of walking for a specific purpose, which by definition is not a gratuitous activity. Walking home from work, walking to the shops, walking to see a neighbour – all give our body some purpose again. The victorious obese person has to relearn how to use their body, which they once considered, and understandably so, as just another weight to carry around and a burden to their freedom.

Leaving obesity behind does not happen by waving a magic wand; it involves re-educating yourself, which takes place in the mind, and you have to want to do it. This requires working on yourself, but it reaps such satisfying results that any concessions are well worth it.

One day a week of pure proteins, three tablespoons of oat bran, flirting with the cold, standing up a lot, walking whenever you can and not taking lifts or escalators – for a person who was once obese but is now stabilizing these are all minor inconveniences compared with the benefits of liberty, dignity and feeling normal again.

Psychological Reinforcement of Stabilization: Three Changes to the Way You Eat

Eat slowly and chew your food thoroughly

It has now been scientifically proven that eating too quickly makes you put on weight. Unbeknown to them, two groups of women were filmed for a British study. The film showed that the group of women of normal weight chewed for twice as long as the group of obese women, which meant that they felt satisfied sooner and had less need to fill up on starchy foods and sugars in the hours following their meal.

There are two ways of feeling satisfied from food: the mechanical satisfaction that you get from filling your stomach; and the real satiety that comes after the food has been digested and gets into your bloodstream and then your brain. People who eat very quickly have to rely on filling their stomachs to calm their greed. This may require enormous quantities of food and explain sleepiness and feeling bloated after meals, which again only goes to prove that too much has been eaten.

On the other hand, a person who eats slowly and chews carefully is allowing time for the calories and nutrients to find their way to the brain, which triggers the signal of feeling satiated. Such a person starts to feel full halfway through a meal and often turns down dessert and cheese.

I realize that it is difficult to totally change this type of firmly rooted behaviour. I also know how exasperating it can be if you are a hare to have to eat alongside a tortoise.

However, if you are an obese person and finding it difficult to stabilize, do not scorn this advice. Accept the idea that a measure as simple as this can make a real difference. Be aware too that deliberately slowing down the speed that you swallow is much easier than it seems. The effort involved in deliberately making sure you chew every mouthful slowly only lasts a few days before it becomes automatic and eventually a habit.

On this subject, I have a story about one of my patients. An Indian gentleman who was once obese, he was cured and stabilized by a guru in a New Delhi ashram who gave him the following piece of advice: 'At each meal, eat and chew as you would normally, but just when you are about to swallow, push the food back to the front of your mouth and chew it for a second time. In two years you will be back at your normal weight again.'

Drink a lot at mealtimes

No one knows exactly where this idea started, but people seem to have the notion that if you want to lose weight you should not drink when you eat. This is not only completely absurd but it flies against the truth. Drinking at mealtimes is good for obese people and for three sound reasons:

- Water is filling and when mixed with food it expands the stomach, producing a feeling of fullness and satisfaction. A wet sponge takes up more space than a dry one.
- Drinking with meals also enables the absorption of solid food to be momentarily interrupted. This pause, as the taste buds are rinsed, slows the meal down, allowing the chemicals that send out messages of satisfaction more time to pass through the blood and reach the brain so that you stop feeling hungry.
- Finally, cold, or even slightly cooled water, lowers the overall temperature of the food in the stomach, which then needs to be warmed up before entering the bloodstream, which takes time and burns up extra calories.

In practice, to take full advantage of all these reasons for drinking water with meals, it is best to drink it cold. Drink a large glass before your meal, another during the meal and one last glass before you leave the table.

Never take second helpings of the same dish

During the Consolidation phase, which is the transition between the weight-loss period and permanent stabilization, the diet opens the door to a number of necessary foods, plus two celebration meals along with the common sense recommendation: 'never take seconds'.

Very obese people, whose weight stabilization is never a certain thing, are well advised to follow this one rule which most naturally thin people do spontaneously. Serve yourself a large portion at the start of the meal knowing that there will be no seconds. You will eat with a better appetite and you can take your time. As soon as you feel tempted to ask for more, you are on dangerous ground. Put your plate down and think about the next course.

Conclusion

What could be easier? Drink when you eat, chew properly so that you can concentrate on all the flavours in your mouth and never take a second helping of the same dish. Simple, to be sure, and effective when applied at the table, the very spot where your high-risk eating habits, which are in part responsible for your obesity in the first place, hold sway. When these measures are followed, they can slowly help tackle the seriously obese person's reckless cravings.

Combined with the other exceptional measures, using the cold and walking with a purpose, specifically intended for the most stubborn cases of obesity, these three measures offer extra rules that while not too difficult to follow are very effective and practical.

A seriously obese person has to understand that they can never hope to permanently stabilize their weight without letting go of a part of themselves, that part which is rooted, through behaviour and through habit, in instability and inevitable failure.

These instructions, which they can depend on, act like beacons on the road to stabilization. They continually confirm the significance, the scope and the permanence of this huge challenge, which is to live comfortably and to eat for the rest of your life, six days out of seven, just like everybody else.

MY PROGRAMME FROM CHILDHOOD THROUGH TO MENOPAUSE

The guiding principle underlying my programme is that in our times it has become difficult to achieve and maintain a normal weight, without some special method.

As I write these lines, in the headquarters and laboratories of the largest food-manufacturing companies there are marketing geniuses, professional psychologists and experts on the deeper motives of human behaviour all working quietly away on whole ranges of snacks, of various shapes and colours, with slogans and advertising campaigns that are so sophisticated that resisting their temptation is virtually impossible.

Alongside this, in other laboratories equally expert researchers and technicians are beavering away to discover and promote methods and appliances whose innovatory features aim to reduce even further the human body's activity and movement. So it is that since the invention of the steam engine, the car, electricity, the telephone, washing machines and spin driers, disposable tissues and nappies, TV remote controls and finally the electric toothbrush, we have been presented with products that according to your point of view either relieve us from or deprive us of a whole array of practical activities and the calories they would be helping us burn up.

This is all to say that every human being living in an elite consumerist society, apart from the few remaining manual workers and professional athletes, has great difficulty in regulating their body weight, yet culturally and socially it has become incorrect to be overweight, both for health reasons and because of prevailing cultural stereotypes that everywhere impose the ideal of being thin.

I designed my programme to confront the way that modern society is drifting in the wrong direction and to provide a programme that could be adapted to every facet of this new disease of modern times.

Up until now, I have presented it in a general way so that its basic structure could be easily understood; and the only parameters given have been for the length of dieting and the amount of weight to be lost. Now it is time to see how this tool can evolve and be adapted for different ages and stages in our lives.

The Dukan Diet in Childhood

The combination of taking less exercise and being bombarded with all kinds of foods has had a pronounced effect on our children. In just one generation, television, computer games and the internet have glued them to their screens, as they snack on a whole array of confectionery, sweets, chewing gum, biscuits and crisps with irresistible flavours promoted by equally irresistible commercials.

The epidemic of American obesity started in the 1960s and took hold of the kids of that generation. Nowadays, those overweight children have become today's fat moms and dads and the USA has the highest rate of obesity in the world.

Paediatricians in my country have already noted the first signs of this cultural invasion. The rate of child obesity in Europe is increasing with American fast foods, pizza, ice cream, fizzy drinks, candy bars, popcorn and breakfast cereals, combined with 'computer game immobility'.

As far as the overweight child is concerned, we should make a distinction between preventive measures for children from families prone to obesity, who very early on show signs of becoming overweight, and curative measures for those children already most at risk from our consumer culture. Never forget that when dealing with overweight children, preventive measures reap the most rewards because once a child becomes overweight they will have to deal with weight control problems for the rest of their life.

So, be well-informed and firm and always try prevention, so that the child avoids becoming overweight and avoids a never-ending and frustrating battle through adulthood.

The child at risk
Generally the child has overweight and easy-going parents, is inactive, loves food, has a big appetite and is chubby from the outset.

For a child, there is certainly no question of starting on a diet and especially not one as structured and effective as my programme. However, help must be given to parents who do not know how to deal with this tendency.

Our advice is clear and simple:

- Never buy or bring home foods that taste of sugar (such as breakfast cereals and juices) except those sweetened with aspartame.
- Absolutely avoid potato crisps, chips and nuts such as peanuts and pistachios.
- Never purchase processed foods for children that are high in sugar and fat.
- Reduce by half or by two-thirds the fats (oil, butter, cream) used in sauces and dressings.

With these few pieces of advice, elementary but effective in the long term, the greatest dangers will be avoided. These measures are non-negotiable because the child's future health, both physical and psychological, is at stake.

An aware and responsible parent will avoid bringing home any and every kind of confectionery, cake, chocolate and ice cream and will reserve them for birthdays, special occasions or rewards. This should be easy enough to do given that nowadays there are so many types of replacement and non-fat products, sugar-free jams, sugar-free chewing gum, flavoured dairy products, low-fat chocolate, yoghurt ice cream etc. Parents can draw on their inventiveness to reduce the oil in salad dressings and the butter on pasta, bread and in sauces for meat, fish and poultry dishes. (See the recipes for sauces and dressings on pages 163–172.)

The overweight child

When dealing with a child under ten who is becoming overweight, parents should adopt a relaxed approach, aiming to stabilize the child's weight at this point so that the nutritional demands for their natural growth will use up the extra pounds. To achieve this, apply the measures mentioned above for three months to correct the balance of fats and sugar in the child's diet.

If their weight continues to go up regardless of these measures, use the Consolidation phase in my programme, with its two celebration meals but without the protein Thursdays, which are too extreme for a child of this age.

If the child is over ten years old and by constitution overweight, it is now possible to try to gradually reduce these extra pounds. Start with the whole Consolidation phase as before, using the day of proteins to keep on track but WITH vegetables. The aim here is to enable the child to lose weight without force or frustration, knowing that they have the great advantage of their growing bodies, which will use up this extra weight for their natural growth.

The Dukan Diet in Adolescence

For a long time, in normal circumstances, adolescence was the time when boys were least likely to become overweight, as it is a time of rapid growth and lots of activity when burning up energy neutralizes any weight gain.

However, it is not the same for adolescent girls, who go through a period of hormonal instability reflected in irregular menstrual periods and weight gain concentrated in the most feminine parts of the body: the thighs, hips or knees. As their bodies change, girls often become emotionally hypersensitive and obsessed with being thin.

The adolescent girl at risk

- If a girl simply tends to be a bit chubby during this stage of irregular periods and noticeable premenstrual syndrome, you should consult your doctor, who can estimate the maturity of her bone structure and how much more growth her body is likely to undergo.
- If the girl is still growing, my Consolidation diet is best suited for this situation and is usually enough to get her weight under control – provided it is followed correctly and includes protein Thursdays.
- If she has finished growing, or she has not lost enough weight following the previous diet, get her to follow the Cruise diet but adapting it for a vulnerable teenager. Whereas adults alternate between pure proteins and pure proteins + vegetables, a teenage girl will always have vegetables with the pure proteins.
- Should her weight gain get worse, from the age of 17 she may follow the full Cruise diet, the one an adult uses, using the 1/1 rhythm, i.e. pure proteins one day then proteins + vegetables the next, until she reaches

her True Weight taking her age into account – but certainly not some self-selected weight termed as an ideal weight as this would be unrealistic or take too long and risk making her body used to a diet that is too restrictive during adolescence.

The obese girl in adolescence

If after the age of 18 a girl is definitely obese, has regular periods and no eating disorders such as bulimia or compulsive eating, she should follow my programme as normal, beginning with three to five days of the Attack diet then moving to the Cruise diet, with an alternating rhythm of one day of pure proteins followed by one day of pure proteins + vegetables.

For adolescent girls, it is even more crucial to consolidate the target weight with the Consolidation diet then move on to stabilization, with its protein Thursdays, no lifts or escalators and three tablespoons of oat bran. If the weight loss was significant, or if there is a past family history of obesity, these three measures should be followed for the appropriate length of time.

The Dukan Diet and Women on the Pill

The new low dosage contraceptive mini-pills have considerably reduced the risk of weight gain associated with the larger doses of earlier birth control pills.

Nevertheless, whatever dosage is used, the first months of taking a contraceptive pill are a time when women put on weight and for anyone who has never had to watch what they eat it is often difficult to get rid of these pounds. This mostly happens at the beginning and gradually lessens over three or four months, a short period during which it is wise to take a few precautions.

Prevention
If you have a personal or family predisposition to putting on weight or are using a high-dose pill, a simple and effective method is to use my permanent Stabilization diet with its protein Thursdays, no lifts or escalators and three tablespoons of oat bran. If this does not work or produce the desired results, follow the complete Consolidation diet with protein Thursdays.

If you are already overweight
- If you are not very overweight, start with the Cruise diet, the 1/1 version (one day proteins followed by one day proteins + vegetables) until you get back down to your normal weight. Then follow the Consolidation diet, five days for every pound lost, followed by the permanent Stabilization diet for at least four months, so that you do not run the risk of regaining the lost weight right away.
- If you are very overweight, follow the entire programme, through all the stages, sticking to protein Thursdays for one year.

The Dukan Diet and Pregnancy

The ideal weight gain during pregnancy (final weight before giving birth) is between 18 and 27 pounds depending on height, age and the number of previous pregnancies. Women predisposed to weight gain may put on a lot more during pregnancy. Thanks to the many different features of my programme's approach, all possibilities can be easily managed.

During pregnancy
- Simple prevention and monitoring. Prevention is the best strategy for women who have already put on too much weight in previous pregnancies, or for women with a history of diabetes or diabetes in their family and also for those who simply want to take care of their figure. These preventive steps can be adopted as soon as possible, and should be followed throughout the entire pregnancy: follow the Consolidation diet but adapt it for pregnancy by incorporating the following changes:
    - eat two portions of fruit per day, instead of one
    - instead of non-fat products use semi-skimmed (less than 2% fat) milk and milk products (yoghurts, cottage cheese etc.)
    - leave out protein Thursdays.
- If you were already overweight before becoming pregnant. This is for women who were already overweight and became pregnant before they could slim down. They may become seriously and worryingly overweight and the solution is to follow my Consolidation diet, which is strengthened by cutting out all starchy foods and the two celebration meals but keeping protein Thursdays.

If clearly obese with a high risk of complications for either the foetus or the mother during pregnancy or during delivery, the Cruise diet can be used, especially at the beginning of the pregnancy. Even the Attack diet may be used at this time, but only with the advice and guidance of a doctor. In such exceptional circumstances, the advantages and disadvantages of such strict dieting have to be weighed up against each other for mother and baby.

After delivery

Now comes the classic situation of trying to get back down to your previous weight by losing a few or a lot of extra pounds. However, every woman should know that it is not always easy or even desirable to try, at all costs, to return to their exact pre-pregnancy weight, which is the same as clinging to what they weighed as a young girl. Based on my experience in this area, I have started applying my own personal calculation for how a woman's weight should change depending on her age and number of pregnancies.

For example, compared with a young (20 years) woman's weight, I consider that between the ages of 20 and 50 the average weight increase is about two pounds for every ten years, plus around four and a half pounds for each child. Therefore, a woman who weighs 7 stone 12 pounds at 20, weighs 8 stone 8 at 25 (including what she has gained from two pregnancies); at 30 she weighs just over 8 stone 9, at 40 she is 8 stone 11, and now at 50 she weighs almost 9 stone.

- Breastfeeding. However much weight you have put on, at this stage it is inconceivable to follow an overly strict diet that would affect the newborn baby's nutrition.

  I recommend eating as if you were simply managing your weight during a normal pregnancy, following the Consolidation diet made easier by:
  - having two portions of fruit per day instead of one
  - using semi-skimmed (less than 2% fat) milk and milk products instead of skimmed 0% fat products
  - leaving out protein Thursdays.
- If you are not breastfeeding. You may start losing weight as soon as you get home from hospital. If your weight gain is normal and a week after the delivery you have between 12 and 16 extra pounds, you can return to your normal weight by following the Cruise diet with a 1/1 alternating rhythm, one day of pure proteins followed by one of proteins + vegetables. Follow this without interruption until you get back down to your desired weight, but do not forget to follow on with the Consolidation diet of five days for every pound lost. Then continue with the permanent Stabilization diet and its three measures: protein Thursdays, no lifts or escalators and oat bran for at least four months.

  If you still have between 22 and 45 extra pounds a week after giving birth, you will have to follow the entire programme with a rapid kick-start of five days on the pure protein Attack diet, moving to the alternating rhythm of the Cruise diet, then the Consolidation diet, finally using over a very long period the permanent Stabilization diet with its three non-negotiable measures: protein Thursdays, no lifts or escalators and oat bran. Keep to this final stage for at least one year, or even longer for women who have not been able to control their weight in the past.

The Dukan Diet and Premenopause and Menopause

The dangers of menopause

Premenopause and the first six months of confirmed menopause is a time of hormonal change, fraught with danger, when women most often put on weight. The body gradually burns up fewer calories with the combined effects of age, reduction in muscle mass and a lowering of thyroid secretion. At the same time, the ovaries stop secreting progesterone, one of their two hormones, creating an imbalance responsible for irregular periods, late periods or a total absence of periods. Progesterone supplements, usually synthetic, are often used to compensate for this change.

The combined effects of these factors cause weight gain, which does not respond to the ordinary eating measures that most women use to control their weight, some more successfully than others.

We are now at the heart of the premenopause, when the ovaries fade away and stop secreting oestrogen, signalled by the start of hot flushes. We have now reached confirmed menopause and if you are using hormone replacement therapy, which now combines progesterone and oestrogen, you will tend to put on even more weight and this will continue while the body adapts to this new treatment but will taper off in a few months.

During this difficult period, which can last two to five years, according to statistics you may put on between 7 and 11 pounds, depending on the kind of replacement therapy being used and how gradual the dosages are. For women prone to gaining weight or who are simply unprepared, this may increase to over 20 or even up to 45 pounds.

Vegetable hormones: an original and natural alternative for women at risk

Much controversy surrounds the risks connected with hormone therapy for the menopause and this has put people off using female hormones. To tackle the difficulties sometimes encountered during the menopause, including hot flushes and alarming weight gain, a totally vegetable-based treatment has been suggested, which is of particular interest to us here.

These natural vegetable substances have a structure so similar to that of female hormones that they can occupy and, partly, replace their receptors. Although less active than female hormones, it has been clinically proven that they give protection from hot flushes. Furthermore, it seems that regular use of the phyto-oestrogens in soya beans, provided they are used in sufficient quantity, enables women, particularly those already overweight or likely to become so, to avoid inevitable menopausal weight gain

However, since phyto-oestrogens are one thousand to two thousand times less powerful than a woman's natural hormones, most doses available in gel or pill form are not high enough to deal with weight risks. According to Japanese research, women in that country do not experience hot flushes and their weight is stable throughout the premenopause and menopause because they regularly eat 200g (7oz) of tofu daily – 200g of tofu is a daily 100mg dose of soya isoflavones, a dose which seems to have the best chance of helping with weight control.

All the authors who have studied the soya bean's nutritional properties insist that, although its protective action very quickly tackles certain menopausal symptoms, such as hot flushes and ageing of the skin, to exploit its preventive effects against breast cancer, osteoporosis and weight gain it has to be used over a long period of time, which alone explains why Asian women have such surprising immunity to these diseases, as they consume a great quantity of soya.

I therefore advise young woman to start eating soya regularly. Not just the sprouts, which do not actively protect you, but the beans themselves or, even better, soya milk and tofu.

Preventive measures
- Normal menopause. When there is no history of abnormal weight gain or dieting but you simply want to be careful, I would advise you, at the first sign of any

premenopause irregularities, to follow the Stabilization diet with its pure protein Thursdays, giving up lifts and escalators and oat bran. In most cases, this will be enough to prevent normal weight gain. You must keep up this defence for the whole, usually chaotic, premenopause phase and continue until the body has fully adapted to the menopause, particularly if you start any hormone replacement therapy when there is the greatest risk of putting on weight.

- Potentially difficult menopause. This is what many women have to contend with if they have always had difficulty maintaining their normal weight and, alone or with the help of their doctor, have contained their tendency to gain pounds. At the first signs of the menopause these women are right to be concerned about habitual weight problems.

If the Stabilization diet is not enough to prevent weight gain, step up a notch and follow the phase three Consolidation diet based on proteins and vegetables, fruit, a portion of wholegrain bread and cheese, two portions of starchy foods per week, the celebration meals and, of course, do not forget the driving power of the pure protein Thursdays.

At certain critical stages of the premenopause, it is vital to step up another notch and follow the phase two Cruise diet, alternating one day of proteins with one day of proteins + vegetables for as long as there is a threat of weight gain, for example when periods become very delayed or virtually absent; when suffering from water retention, various swellings, bloated stomach, heavy legs, fingers so puffy you cannot remove your rings, headaches; and during the first three critical months of hormone replacement therapy. Normally, this diet is enough to maintain an effective defence.

If you are already overweight

- A recent weight gain. If no precautions have been taken and weight has recently been gained, but is not yet threatening, I recommend starting with three days of my Attack diet followed by the Cruise diet, alternating one day of pure proteins with one day of proteins + vegetables. Once you are back to your correct weight, use the protective Consolidation diet and its natural sequel, the permanent Stabilization diet, which you should follow until your body is perfectly used to your hormone replacement therapy, i.e. at least six months.

- Overweight for quite a while. If you already have a tendency to gain weight, or have been overweight or obese for a long period of time, you might want to avoid starting hormone replacement therapy for the time being. Or worse, if you have already started a treatment and have seen your weight explode, I would advise you to follow the Attack diet to the letter, starting with five days of pure proteins, or even seven days if you have put on a significant amount of weight. Then move on to the Cruise diet, the 5/5 version, alternating five days of pure proteins with five days of proteins + vegetables, or use a 1/1 version if the weight gain is not so great or you are able to lose it more easily. Once you reach your desired weight, continue with the Consolidation diet for as many days as our rule requires, i.e. five days for every pound lost. Finally, keep to the permanent Stabilization diet for the rest of your life.

The Dukan Diet and Giving Up Smoking

Breaking the habit and putting on weight

Many people hesitate, justifiably so, to give up smoking for fear that they will put on weight. There are also people who, having managed to give up smoking, see their weight shoot up in reaction, so they start smoking again in the mistaken belief that by doing so they will lose this weight, only to sacrifice the marvellous benefits of their hard work and compound their problems.

You need to realize that the extra pounds that come from giving up smoking are due to two related factors.

The ex-smoker needs to find other forms of oral satisfaction, other odours, flavours and gestures that are different but similar to those of smoking, categorized by paediatricians and psychologists as 'oral stage sensations', in reference to the oral stage in early infancy described by Freud and his successors. From this need to find sensations similar to smoking comes the need to put something in your mouth, the need to nibble between meals on snacks with all kinds of intense and pleasant flavours, which increase your calorie intake.

While the need for new sensations brings extra

calories, other calories are accumulating that the nicotine previously burnt up.

The combination of these sensory and metabolic factors means that ex-smokers can put on an average of ten and sometimes as many as 20 or 30 pounds depending on predisposition and whether they were addicted, heavy smokers.

Weight gained while giving up tobacco is virtually locked in and will not disappear spontaneously if you start smoking again. So it is vital to hold on to the extraordinary achievement of overcoming dependency on a drug as dangerous as tobacco.

Remember, too, that the risk of putting on weight through giving up smoking is a one-off thing and limited to six months, so the effort required to fight any weight gain is also limited in time. Once past this period, your metabolism returns to normal, reactions to oral satisfaction diminish and weight control becomes much easier.

How a normal-weight smoker can avoid putting on extra pounds

Let's look now at a smoker of normal weight, who has no personal predisposition or family history of weight gain and has never dieted in the past.

The best strategy for a light smoker, who smokes fewer than ten cigarettes a day or who does not inhale, is to follow the permanent Stabilization diet with its pure protein Thursdays, stairs only and oat bran for six months.

269

For a heavy smoker, who gets through over 20 cigarettes a day, the Consolidation diet is better and should be followed to the letter in the first four months after giving up smoking, followed by the phase four permanent Stabilization diet for the next four months.

How a smoker with a predisposition to weight gain can avoid putting on extra pounds

If you are in this category or have other risk factors such as diabetes, respiratory or heart problems, my advice is that as soon as you give up smoking you should begin under the protection of phase two of my programme, the Cruise diet 1/1 version, i.e. alternating one day of proteins with one day of proteins + vegetables, and so on for the first full month, which is precisely when the risk of putting on weight is the greatest. Then move on to the Consolidation diet for five months, and afterwards use the permanent Stabilization diet for a minimum of six months.

Obesity and quitting smoking

There is here a very high health risk as putting on any extra pounds will aggravate an already dangerous situation. This is difficult as the pre-existing obesity shows that gaining weight is easy and that smoking and nicotine did nothing to keep off the pounds. We may face the risk of an explosion in snacking and cravings for oral satisfaction.

Nevertheless, the benefits are equal to the difficulty because giving up smoking combined with weight loss in an obese person frees the body from the double threat of cardiovascular disease and lung cancer.

This extremely hard and treacherous road necessitates very strong motivation and both medical and psychological support from a doctor, who may prescribe tranquillizers or even anti-depressants to lessen the shock from the change in these two major behaviour patterns.

In such urgent cases, I prescribe my programme in its strictest version, starting with the pure proteins Attack phase for five to seven days, followed by a Cruise diet alternating one day of pure proteins with one day of proteins + vegetables, then moving on to Consolidation whose length is calculated according to the rule of five days for every pound lost. Finally, and most importantly, go into the last phase of my programme, the permanent Stabilization phase, and its trio of preventive measures: protein Thursdays, no lifts or escalators, and three tablespoons of oat bran, to be followed for life.

How to lose weight if you have already given up smoking
Here, the damage is done and was not avoided in time. You have completely achieved your goal of giving up smoking but have gained extra weight in doing so; it is important to avoid at any price the temptation to start smoking again.

This situation is quite similar to being typically overweight, and can be tackled by using the whole Dukan Diet in its most powerful form: five days of the Attack phase with five days of pure proteins, followed by a Cruise phase alternating one day of pure proteins with one day of proteins + vegetables. Then follow the Consolidation phase for five days for every pound lost. Finally, and most importantly, go into the last phase of my programme, the permanent Stabilization diet and its trio of preventive measures – protein Thursdays, no lifts or escalators, and three tablespoons of oat bran – and stick to this for at least eight months, or for the rest of your life if you have put on a lot of weight (over 30 pounds) and if you used to smoke more than one pack of cigarettes a day.

BEING ACTIVE:
THE ESSENTIAL CATALYST

Dear reader,

If you REALLY want to lose weight,

If you REALLY want to never again put weight back on,

you must TOTALLY change how you view exercise.

This chapter gives you the means to increase twofold the effectiveness and permanence of the results achievable with my diet programme.

The book you are holding tells the story of the path my career as a doctor took.

In 1970, I created the foundation of my diet. Back then, when losing weight was all that mattered, it offered 72 high protein foods – an Attack diet with brilliant but short-lived results.

Very early on, I added to it the 28 vegetables to turn it into a more stable Cruise diet and all these prescribed foods formed the basis of my 100 Foods.

In the 1980s, I included the Consolidation phase so that once dieters went back to eating normally, better protection would be provided for the results they had achieved.

Then in the 1990s, I added the most innovative section to this diet: the permanent Stabilization phase to shore up over the very long term the weight loss that had been achieved.

By 2000, I considered this programme as quite complete. It was handed over as it was to my readers and medical peers without any inkling that it would encounter such a huge success. Today this book has been read by several million people. It features on many websites, forums and blogs, it has been translated in many countries, has been greeted with such enthusiasm and many men and women have done me the honour of making it their own that this book and the method it contains no longer just belongs to me. In short, and I say this most sincerely, this book belongs to you, especially as it is no longer quite mine. So many anonymous ordinary people have passed my message on to others that I feel a great responsibility towards these readers.

It was for this very reason that I asked my publisher to hand me back the mic, as I had something to say and write that is vitally important. And it is this message that is the raison d'être for this chapter and which alone should give you the means to increase twofold the effectiveness and permanence of the results achievable with my programme.

Since this book first appeared more than fifteen years have passed. The world has become a harsher place and at a rate that outstrips our search for remedies to deal with all the problems this creates. One of these problems is being overweight, and for me this is one of the most significant pointers flagging up just how difficult it is to find fulfilment in today's world. Our world can offer a way of living that is both rich and stimulating, but also one where instinct and nature have got lost along the way.

We have created this world – it's our world and the world to which we have become accustomed and could not now live without. Yet it is a world that does harm. And you who are reading my book are amongst those who can bear witness to this harm because you eat to do yourselves good!

Over the past fifteen years there has been an ever growing increase in weight and obesity problems. Don't misunderstand me; it's not simply that with each passing year there are more overweight people. But rather the extent of the problem becomes ever greater, so that each year as we climb up the obesity ladder the rungs move even higher. This means that not only are we failing to make the right choices, BUT WE ARE MAKING THE WRONG CHOICES.

So it is essential that a solution is found that is sufficiently convincing to win over doubters and create a consensus so that we can bring together all the experience, expertise, resources and funding that we need to be able to better tackle this societal problem, which the World Health Organization has ranked as being the sixth scourge of humanity.

And it is the reason for this chapter.

The Limitations of Just Dieting

In this book, including the version you have here, my readers have found my diet with its four phases, each one broken down into its foods with a road map to explain them, and the 100 foods, of which 72 are protein foods and 28 are vegetables.

I've already told you that to date more than 3.2 million people have bought the book you're holding. My publisher assures me that every book sold is read on average by 3 people, which means that almost 10 million men and women have read this book.

I don't know how many of those people who bought the book then went on to follow the diet. I know even less about how many achieved their True Weight after following it. Nor do I know – and this is what is most important to me – having achieved their True Weight, how many managed to stabilize it despite life's many trials and tribulations. However, I do know two things of which I am certain and which I can guarantee you:

- Firstly, I do not know anyone who has not lost weight having followed this diet as it is prescribed. Their results may vary depending on their gender, age, how long they were overweight, hereditary factors or the number of diets already tried. But anyone who has followed the diet has lost weight; at their own speed, but they have lost weight.
- I also know that a considerable number of the people who have read and used my method have consolidated

and stabilized their weight in the long term, i.e. for over three years. I know this for a fact as my readers regularly write and tell me.

Nevertheless, I also receive letters and emails from people who, having lost weight, followed their Consolidation phase and started their permanent Stabilization phase, manage to keep going for a while but then lose their way and some of the weight they had lost goes back on. Why? I know about all the reasons for such setbacks as I come across them in my consultations. I have analyzed and categorized them thus:

- Some people did not have the motivation, trigger or even the inclination to read the book and start the programme. The book is still lying on a bookshelf waiting for whatever it is that will get them going.
- Others have read it and started the programme but stopped because they did not have the motivation or energy required to attain their True Weight.
- Others at certain ages or critical times in their lives found themselves up against physiological resistance from their hormones, ovaries or thyroid, or they have suffered depression and their medication has had an impact on their weight. With all these difficulties you are vulnerable to stagnation plateaux, brief or lengthy, which without support undermine resistance, mistakes happen and the dieting gets abandoned.
- The same goes for people who have tried too many

diets without achieving results or stabilization, diets that are too restrictive, too tiring, too lacking in certain nutrients, too inconsistent, which do not work or are not followed properly, the very diets that lead to repeated weight regain – i.e. bad diets. Here we also find people who, despite not overeating, still gain weight easily because of hereditary factors and genes. For all of them, the struggle is hard and the resistance greater.

- Finally, and this is the biggest group, people who while losing weight, in whatever phase, encounter personal difficulties: disappointment in love, divorce, overwork, workplace problems or any one of life's many other painful events. When in such turmoil, very few can resist the urge to reach out for food as a 'comfort', especially those vulnerable to weight problems who eat as a natural defence against stress and lack of pleasure and security, a habit acquired early on in childhood.

It was for such difficult cases, these high-risk dieters and anyone coping with life's troubles, that eventually I concluded that prescribing my diet on its own was not enough. So I opened a second front to step up the attack and, with a pincer movement, trap my old enemy who eludes capture at every opportunity.

Before getting to the core of this chapter I would like to start by summarizing how my programme works. Its success is based on the combination of ten winning factors – plus one extra:

1. The effectiveness of proteins.
2. The speed with which the Attack phase starts off.
3. Total freedom regarding quantities; avoiding the frustration of feeling racked by hunger.
4. The simplicity of its instructions: 100 foods, 72 protein foods and 28 of vegetables.
5. A strong, firm internal framework: the four phases are structured and signposted, from the strictest to the most flexible, each one with its own purpose, rhythm and bench marks.
6. An educational side which teaches you about weight loss while you are losing weight. The order in which foods are introduced records in your body's memory their relative importance, starting off with what is vital (proteins) then essential (vegetables), necessary (fruits), important (wholemeal bread), useful (starchy foods), rewarding (cheese) and pleasure-giving (celebration meals).
7. Stabilization and the absolute importance given to this phase: two out of the four stages, consolidation and permanent stabilization (the latter lasting for the rest of your life), aim to ensure you not only lose weight but are 'cured of being overweight'.
8. An approach that through a human face, empathy and active support helps you manage your motivation, pleasure and lack of pleasure and what is going on in your mind.

But this method lacked three elements for it to offer a real counterattack and stem the worrying escalation in the weight problem battle:

1. **A personalized approach.** When dealing with weight problems this is of paramount importance. For the person losing weight, it offers them assurance that they are not alone. Personalizing means bringing in a 'project manager' who is capable of examining how a person is coping with 'their' foods, their weak and strong points; and, after collecting all this information, of devising an action plan that suits the individual's personality, which will then, by definition, be infinitely more effective. But above all it means knowing how to help that person by using their strengths to correct their weaknesses so that after losing weight they avoid finding themselves back in the very situations that made them put it on.

2. **Daily monitoring.** This is the simplest and most effective way of lessening the unpleasantness of dieting and the inevitable frustrations it imposes. Being monitored, receiving precise and firm instructions from someone who is authoritative and in whom you trust means you are better equipped to resist temptation and make the right choices.

   Being monitored means knowing that you have to report back about your dieting, your lapses, your difficulties, doubts and failings. Being monitored means not being left on your own to face one of the most dangerous dieting traps, the moment when without any apparent reason your weight inevitably stagnates.

3. Lastly, and this is the purpose of this chapter, a final point that is perhaps more crucial than all the others: EXERCISE.

Exercise is the second general in the army, just as important as dieting in this fight against weight problems.

I have to admit that if, like everyone else, I have always known that exercise plays a key part in leading a healthy life and keeping weight under control, I belong to a generation for whom being active was so natural and obvious that I never felt the burning need to prove it. When I was a child, AIDS did not exist and people passed away mysteriously from cancer. What haunted people back then was the fear of paralysis. All mothers lived in fear of polio and 'wheelchairs'. My mother loved me enough to have passed on to me both this anxiety and the importance of being physically active. And so walking, running, swimming, dancing, jumping for joy and singing at the top of my voice became ingrained in my emotional memory as being the natural ingredients of life.

When I was a student, my first locum job was in the old part of Montparnasse, a lively, colourful part of Paris where my home visits were mostly to apartment blocks with no lifts, so I had to cheerfully climb up many, many stairs.

Being physically active has always been part of my nature and culture and, because of this, I must confess that it took me quite a while to realize the extent to which being inactive and reluctant to make any physical effort is a dreadful hindrance to rapid, effective and long-lasting weight loss with low frustration.

It was a trivial incident that brought this home to me. I was queuing in a Spanish travel agency where three employees were dealing with customers at the counter. All had comfortable chairs on casters which meant they could move about without getting up. Two of them seemed to enjoy propelling themselves around, sometimes fetching files that were several metres away. The third employee always got up and whether it was pure coincidence or thermodynamics he was slim whereas the other two, despite their youth, already had a paunch.

From that day, this ordinary scene changed the way I approached the fight against weight problems. I suddenly realized how crucial it had become to incorporate exercise into my programme. Not by giving simple common-sense advice as everyone involved in the field does, but by recommending and structuring it with as much force and determination as I did with the diet. I told myself that if I, a hardened warrior who had devoted his career to fighting weight problems, had not fully understood the extent to which we are currently neglecting our bodies, I could imagine how much my readers might also have underestimated its importance.

Because, if it is true that we all know in theory that being active burns up calories, this is purely on an intellectual level and has not been transformed into core instinctive conviction. In fact we all do know it, but nobody believes it, or at the very least nobody believes it enough to deem it as important as giving up food.

So I started not just recommending exercise, as I had always done, I PRESCRIBED it just like medicine.

However, in practice what seems so simple comes up against the problem of its very simplicity – it is as if breathing were being prescribed! First of all, when I ask the following straightforward question, 'Do you take exercise?', I get only vague and evasive answers: 'I walk a bit like anyone else' or 'When you've got children you can't help but be active'. But when I probe deeper a very clear division emerges between two types of exercise: exercise with a purpose, when we have to make an effort and move around to achieve practical goals in our daily lives, and 'being active for its own sake' as dictated by our prevailing cultural attitudes to remain beautiful, toned, slim and healthy, attitudes that make us feel guilty and take out that gym subscription, although we still take the lift up to the gym instead of walking up the stairs. When you realize that people pay to use stepping machines, which are nothing more than steps in gadget form, you can see the paradox.

The problem of taking exercise raises a problem about our society. Our economic models are based on progress, and technology advocates eliminating physical effort. How can we believe in the virtues of exercising for a purpose in our daily lives when half of the patents for new inventions in the world are for methods and machines that aim to reduce pure physical effort and gain time, two ingredients that when combined lead to stress and weight problems?

Moreover, walking is almost as basic as breathing, so much a part of man's nature and human condition that it is hard enough to understand its 'therapeutic' value let alone how it can help us slim.

Finally, it is not sophisticated or technical enough for doctors to bother with, and when I talk of doctors I include myself here. For years, I kept to sound advice, especially regarding walking, but without risking the ridicule of formally writing out a prescription. I thought that patients had not come to see a doctor with umpteen qualifications and years of experience, a specialist in nutrition, to be given a prescription for walking or exercise. How wrong could I be!

As we have come this far together, I am going to try to get you to come a bit further so that you fully understand the decisive challenge involved in adopting this new concept of being 'vitally active' – PRESCRIBED EXERCISE (PE). To do this I will pose two simple, concrete questions and give a totally unambiguous reply:

Does exercise make you lose weight?
After losing weight is exercise vital for stabilizing your weight?
The reply is an overwhelming YES to both questions.

Now let's look at the evidence.

Exercise makes you lose weight

If you open and close your eyes, simply fluttering your eyelids like this makes you burn up energy. Hardly anything, of course, but energy nonetheless that can be measured in millicalories. The same applies if you think or recall something. More so if you think, reflect and solve a problem. Much more if you lift one arm and twice as much if you lift both.

By standing up, you immediately increase calorie-combustion as it forces the body's three biggest muscle groups to contract: the quadriceps, stomach and buttock muscles. Everything you do uses up calories. So far do you agree with me?

Let's continue. Step outside your front door. Let's imagine that you live on the fourth floor. By not taking the lift you will use six calories walking down to the street. You have forgotten something and are in a rush so you run back up the stairs burning off 14 calories then another six walking down again: 26 calories, gone in a trice.

Let's move on. It is lunchtime. You have worked for four hours seated in front of your computer. You have been breathing, your heart has been beating and your blood circulating. Simply keeping your body going, in contact with the world, uses up one calorie per minute. Moreover, during these four hours you have carried out your work tasks and moved your arms and legs, another 15 calories gone. Your legs now feel numb so you want to get up and walk; you go out.

And now, to your great surprise I am going to ask you to walk FOR ONE HOUR! Oh, I realize this is not easy. And why walk when it is possible not to walk? And apart from anything else this is an hour out of your work time. Let's imagine that you agree. If you walk without pushing yourself but without dawdling either you will use up 300 calories in one hour. All in all, at this precise moment since opening your front door you have used up around 340 calories. A clear, defined amount but for you it is an abstract figure, disconnected from your intuitive perception. This is true.

If you lived in a different world, the world of primitive man, the hunter-gatherer, dictated by shortages directly dependent on the natural environment, things would be quite different. In such a world, where you would have to use up energy to hunt and capture your food, walking for pleasure would carry a risk, that of needlessly drawing on your vital, strategic and precious reserves. A limited risk if just a one-off event, but considerable if you took it into your head to do this every single day. You can see how incredibly important exercise is for managing our human energy reserves. These reserves are precisely what you are trying to get rid of and what these first humans held on to for their very survival. Here you have put your finger on the crux of why it is so difficult to lose weight and how much exercise will help and how.

Let's come back to you. If you are reading this book it is probably because you are overweight. If this is so, each pound of fat that you are carrying on your hips and thighs if you are a gynoid shape, or on your bust and tummy if an android shape, each one of these pounds that you hate so much stores a little over 4,000 calories. Scientifically this means that you need only walk one hour a day, five days a week, for three weeks to get rid of one pound. Take an example: 300 calories x 15 days = 4,500 calories = one pound of your fat. And without changing what you eat. This hour of walking could alone sort out your weight problems. Too good to be true! I can already hear all the objections coming thick and fast. Who has an hour a day, five times a week? How can you fit this into a busy working life?

I agree that we all lead busy lives, so I am going to show you how to fit exercise into your schedule and use it in conjunction with the diet. What I am trying to do here is to highlight exercise's impressive firepower, which is and always has been available to us. Even better – it is a strength that we carry in us and on us. So then why haven't we drawn upon this immense resource earlier, other than in the form of simple common-sense advice, which de facto prevented it from being at all effective? Because once you see – and I've been working in the field for many years – all the effort put into advocating calorie restriction with its high failure rates, you realize how messages informing people about how effective exercise can be must have been badly communicated, or they simply just didn't get across.

Is being active more unpleasant or difficult than dieting? The answer is NO!

Provided you are convinced that it works. It seems that up until now, for the vast majority of those proposing and using diets, the only way to guarantee that you would lose weight was to diet and restrict access to food – exercise was only there so you would have a clear conscience, protect your muscle mass and tone your body. This is why I decided to channel my efforts into getting the message across by making it part of my system. Like everyone else in the field I devised my method around a diet programme. And precisely because it is so successful, I want to add to it what I consider to be no more and no less than a second engine. Because losing weight has a psychological cost, even for people who are completely successful. It is hard to confront who you are; it is an enriching experience, success brings you purpose, meaningful self-actualization, renewed self-esteem. BUT there is also the commitment and the battle, for which you need preparation, supervision, a support structure, a proven and reliable method and care, and vigilance at every moment.

A battle against oneself, but also against other people: against those who would also like to take up the challenge but haven't yet found the impetus and have a bad conscience as they watch others struggle, those inventors of the phrase 'Go on just this once', you know what I mean! A struggle too against our prevalent culture, which promotes consumption; against manufacturers who find it easier to sell rich, fatty and sugary comfort foods rather than what is good for us; against the advertising industry, which comes up with those 'killer' (in every sense of the word) words, slogans and images! Moreover, if my method has so many supporters, who after benefiting from it have made a point of spreading the word, defending it and promoting it, I have a duty to open up what I consider to be a second bridgehead in the fight against weight problems. And it is intended for those men and women who are either struggling or vulnerable and do not have sufficient energy or courage to enter into open conflict with themselves – so that they can lose weight knowing how much this weight loss they so desire will be a help to them both morally and physically.

So I decided to make known what has seemed to me for several years now to be the missing or weak link when battling against weight problems, which is realizing that being active and taking exercise is not just relatively effective but totally effective. I wanted to make a clean break with the vague and uncertain prevailing cultural views that in theory recognize the role exercise plays without in practice providing confirmation.

It seems as if this pussyfooting is typical of the societies we live in, which promote two contradictory commands. On the one hand 'you won't be active', so here are all sorts of instruments created to avoid any needless effort, down to electric toothbrushes. For a long time now robots, mechanization and various methods of transport have lightened our load, every day eroding a little further our movement and how we most naturally express our human nature. On the other hand 'you will be active': the culture of sport, health, anti-ageing, gyms and this paradoxical return to 'machines to make us active' – exercise bikes, treadmills, etc.

Between these two extremes are all sorts of activities that flag up this contradiction.

Exercise helps us control pleasure and lack of pleasure

I am now going to ask you to follow me into unusual territory, into life's inner depths, to the place where your first decisions come into being, the place where your reasons for living and not dying take root. This may all seem very far removed from mundane weight problems; in fact, as you will see, it gets right to the very nub. Come on, follow me and you will not regret it.

If you are overweight, you probably realize that it was not hunger that made you eat and put on those extra pounds. Nowadays, where we live, very few people really go hungry. Today people only put on weight because they eat more than their biological requirements; they eat more than they need to satisfy their hunger. The woman who eats too much, at the same time cursing the extra pounds that are the outcome, is not after nutrition. She eats while driven by a need greater than her fear of becoming fat. So what exactly is she looking for? What she is trying to do, and often without even realizing it, is to create pleasure with something tangible to compensate for not getting enough pleasure in her daily life. Or she wants to neutralize some pain or there is too much stress blocking her horizons. Generally this is how people put on weight.

The difficulty is that in order to lose weight you have to do the opposite: not only stop using food to make up for whatever is missing on other levels but go without, stop eating what you want, in short, create an absence of pleasure, frustration.

So how can you possibly lose weight and keep it off permanently by going against what you are searching for, in a confused way, which is finding pleasure in food, pleasure that is life's driving force and so vital and so essential you will sacrifice your figure, beauty, powers of seduction and sometimes even your health for it. How can a woman, who day after day has sought pleasure in food, suddenly turn her back on all this and follow a slimming diet? This contradiction explains why it is so difficult to lose weight and so easy to put it back on.

And yet it is possible, there is a path, seldom if ever used. This path I am talking of is a narrow ridge between two chasms: on the one side you do nothing and suffer in consequence and on the other you do the wrong thing and fail. The ridge path – the one that enables you to lose weight without regaining it – is the one I call 'being cured of being overweight'. To understand and explore it together, let's open up the bonnet and inspect 'life's engine'.

Around the fifth week of pregnancy, inside the mother's womb, inside the frail embryo that the fertilized egg has turned into, a cerebral centre appears which sends out the first beats of autonomous life and continues doing this until the moment of death. What is this life beat? It is the programming and energy etched into every living creature, so obvious and so vital to the creature that it feels no need to seek it out or even be aware of it. Let's call this centre life's pulsating heart. When it sends out beats, we feel a powerful urge to embrace life and all our actions focus on protecting and promoting life: eating, drinking, sleeping, reproducing, playing, hunting, keeping our bodies working, keeping safe, belonging to a group, making sure we remain in it and find our best place in it according to our abilities.

Each living species works in its own particular way to ensure its survival. We humans have evolved to survive in a human environment. If we follow our behaviour tutors naturally and spontaneously, we improve our chances of survival and our reward is that nice, fulfilling feeling we call pleasure. This is why we experience pleasure when our body is dehydrated and we drink or when our cells have run out of fuel and we eat. Everything that makes survival easier generates pleasure and anything that thwarts it reaps the opposite. Everything we do, we do either to gain pleasure or to avoid the absence of pleasure.

But that is not all; there is far more surprising and even crucial information to come, so please follow me because it will help you to manage your life better. Behind this nice feeling of pleasure, another far more vital 'food' is weaving its way like an invisible partner. Along with pleasure, it enters the brain's neurological pathways;

here pleasure becomes this nice feeling while the other continues on its journey until it reaches the pulsating heart that sends out our life force. This secret passenger has a fundamental role: to get to life's pulsating heart and recharge it with energy to strengthen it and keep it sending out our life force.

To recap, life's pulsating heart beats out our urge and need to live. The life force produced expresses itself through actions and behaviour that seek out and harvest pleasure. And accompanying the feeling of pleasure, a special 'food' comes back to the pulsating heart so that it continues to pulsate. It is in fact a feedback loop, as we so often see in living creatures, but this one is right at the very top of the hierarchy controlling life.

Often confused with pleasure, which is more obvious and masks its partner with its conspicuous pleasantness, this neurological food is of paramount importance. Strangely enough, as far as I know this vital substance has no name. I have called it 'bene-satisfaction' to combine in a single name the dual notion of satisfaction and benefit.

You must be wondering why we have taken such a long detour to justify using exercise to fight weight problems. Firstly, to make you realize that eating is, along with drinking and breathing, what is most necessary for life and is therefore one of the most efficient sources of 'bene-satisfaction'.

You can easily understand how, faced with the struggles of daily existence, many men and women do not manage to get enough of this precious 'bene-satisfaction' without which life's pulsating heart slows down, impoverishing their quality of life. When we reach this point, survival's strident sirens start to blast out, forcing us to get some. And then when this still does not happen life's pulsating heart in turn stops sending out its beats, the desire for life fades away then stops and, as has become so common today, we fall into depression, our primary consciousness obviously failing as our lust for life is lost.

And in this often subconscious, sometimes urgent quest, the easiest and most readily accessible way to get it is quite simply to eat: putting something in our mouths, swallowing, digesting it to feed ourselves and using it to produce contentment, something pleasant and reassuring that up until now we have been confusing with pleasure. Cerebral imagery allows us to visualize the effects of any human behaviour, and the one most charged with emotions, the one which triggers the most intense intra-cerebral fireworks, is eating pleasant foods. As far as neurological impact and production of pleasure go, eating is almost as intense as having an orgasm but it has the added advantage of lasting longer. This is the reason why, in a frustrating environment, it is so easy to put on weight and so difficult to lose it by restricting what we can eat, because eating is our chief source of 'bene-satisfaction'. Here is a striking anecdote about an experiment that has been carried out time and again in all animal physiology laboratories. Place a calibrated rat inside a traditional cage where it is fed from a dish that is always kept full and leave it alone. The rat will eat as much as it wants, stopping once it feels full. If a painless clamp is then placed on the end of its tail, which encumbers the rat as it has to carry it around, the rat will become obese within six weeks. It compensates: protecting itself from this lack of pleasure by counterbalancing it with pleasure – it creates something positive to neutralize the negative.

Let's come back to exercise and how it controls pleasure and 'bene-satisfaction'. If I took this detour advancing such lengthy arguments it is because nowadays exercise is completely undervalued. For most of us it has become a burden, a chore, toil to be avoided. However, for anyone who wants to lose weight it is quite the opposite: exercise can and must become their principal, most powerful ally and friend.

If those people who put on weight overeat knowing full well that doing so will make them overweight then it is because they want to create some 'bene-satisfaction', as without it their life's engine may get jammed up. This usually happens to men and women particularly prone to comfort eating; for them, more than for anyone else, exercise plays a key role in modifying their relation to pleasure and lack of pleasure.

What I am asking you to do is to make an effort to change the way you view exercise. As simple, natural and obvious as using your body may seem, it is this element alone which has to radically change the direction from which we battle against weight problems. Above all, please trust me, I promise you that you will have no regrets.

The Diet's Effectiveness is Greatly Strengthened by Exercise

To gradually reduce the volume or weight of a container you have two alternatives: you fill it up less or you empty it more; just as with business stock you can choose between buying less or selling more. The same logic applies to slimming. You have two methods of 'equal' importance: either you reduce your intake – you eat less and fewer rich foods – or you use up more energy, by being more active and burning up more calories. Ideally you will combine the two. Following the same diet, the more active you are, the more weight you will lose.

Exercise Reduces the Frustration of Dieting

The more active you are and the more calories you burn up, the less you need to limit what you eat and the less you suffer. You absolutely have to get into your mindset that there is an energy conversion principle here between food and exercise.

Exercise Generates Pleasure

Sufficient muscular activity on warm muscles triggers endorphin secretion, a chemical mediator produced in the central nervous system that gives us a feeling of exhilaration. To produce it, a certain amount of muscular training is required, but once you start producing endorphins and once the active body is producing pleasure, being overweight is no longer a long-term problem. One of my patients pointed out to me that she had never managed to fall in love with a diet but that she had become completely hooked on exercise, 'addicted'. In her case I am convinced she will have no trouble keeping at the weight she got down to. One of my slogans – it applies to any activity, action or behaviour but in particular to shedding and gaining weight – explains why:

Anything you do without pleasure annoys
Anything you do with suffering destroys.

Exercise, Unlike Dieting, Enables You to Lose Weight Without Developing Resistance

Here we touch on one of the crucial points when we battle against weight problems. We all know that the more you diet, the more resistant you become to dieting and the harder it becomes to lose weight. Our species came into being at a time when you had to fight to win your food, so fat reserves were the best guarantee of survival. We have been programmed to resist wasting calories and to treasure our fat reserves. Nowadays, we live with abundance and are surrounded by food, but our genes and the way our bodies are programmed have not changed one iota – our bodies are still as viscerally attached to their fat reserves. When the body experiences any weight loss it sees this as dangerous plundering, which it is programmed to repel. How does it do this? It has two options: either by economizing, using up less energy, or by raiding its own reserves. Accordingly the more diets you try the more your body learns to resist; this manifests itself in slower weight loss and the slower the weight loss becomes, the greater the risk of you losing heart and failing.

This type of situation gives rise to the greatest danger in a diet: the stagnation plateau, a period when although still following the diet to the letter you fail to lose any weight. If there is nothing quite as rewarding and encouraging as seeing the pounds slip away, there is nothing as testing as watching your scales fail to deliver the reward you long for. Weight stagnation, when long-lasting and undeserved, is responsible for the highest diet failure rates.

However, and this is crucial, although your body can adapt to reduced calorie intake and dieting it is not equipped to resist calories being burned through exercise. It is not programmed for it. You can burn up 350 calories by gently jogging for an hour every day for months on end and you will also use up the same number of calories. But if you cut out 350 calories from your food intake, within a few weeks your body will have become used to this and you will stop losing weight and then you will have to cut out 500 calories or give up calorie-counting. So the best way of avoiding the disastrous effects of resistance to a succession of diets is to combine dieting with exercise.

Exercise Means You Can Lose Weight and Be Toned

Even for overweight people whose skin is stretched by the fat underneath, well maintained muscle structure makes them look more toned. At the same weight, a trained and muscular body looks more toned, radiant and younger too. You can be proud of your outer appearance, of how others see you and of how you see yourself.

For Long-term Stabilization Exercise is Indispensable

Being active means you do not have to rely so much on restricting what you eat, which in the long term is frustrating. For example, a 20-minute walk cancels out a glass of wine or three squares of chocolate – they are neutralized. We all know that the effort we are willing to make to slim is only possible if it is time-limited, targeted and defined. Once your True Weight has been attained it is time to move on to consolidation then stabilization, which involves opening the way to new foods, so that eating is more spontaneous and less supervised.

Yet from experience we know that life's ups and downs can throw the best established routines into confusion, especially as at such vulnerable times we seek comfort in the most comforting of comfort foods. Taking enough exercise uses up calories and often provides pleasure, which actually means that you can eat more. Exercise allows you to more easily absorb any 'wild lapses and collapses', any 'moments of madness' by burning them up in the 'heat of action', thereby lessening their impact and your feelings of guilt. What is more, exercise enables you to maintain a rhythm, a state of mind, pride in yourself and your body, which stop you from going adrift.

And really, really important is the large-scale endorphin secretion that exercise releases in fit individuals; through the neurological pleasure it creates, exercise reduces the equally neurological need to find solace in eating, in artificial, 'manufactured' pleasure. Depressed women desperate to lose weight throw some light on this. In the short term they manage to follow a diet, provided it is totally structured with enough support. However, keeping this effort up is impossible, especially once the results have been achieved. For as long as they are depressed and 'not happy enough' they automatically revert to comfort eating, their antidote to unhappiness. For them, and even more so for people who are not depressed, finding pleasure in being active while burning up the calories is *the* best way of protecting weight loss.

Exercise Enables You to Break Through a 'Stagnation Plateau'

In my 40-odd years working as a nutritionist, what I have particularly noticed is that the proportion of patients I term as 'difficult cases' and resistant to dieting is outstripping the number of straightforward cases. Who are they? They are mostly women over forty and they fit into one or more of these four categories:

- Women who have a long history of dieting. I love it when, as soon as they are seated in my surgery they say with a knowing smile: 'Doctor, I have to tell you that I have already tried every diet!'

- Often women with a major family history, mothers who come to consultations with an already corpulent child and who themselves have a mother, father, aunts and uncles who are stout and very often diabetic.

- And of course, very stout, obese people who are so overweight that this is impossible to completely reverse. Surprisingly, they are not the most adversely affected by their extra weight. Often I find them to be less determined than those 'almost perfect' dieters desperate to shed the few pounds that are torturing them.

- Finally, almost always people who lead a confirmed sedentary lifestyle, who experience modern times as all hustle and bustle and with the accumulation of chores and fatigue are allergic to any additional effort.

It is these people who have become resistant to diets and who, when they decide to try a new one, know that they are vulnerable. They go for it wholeheartedly and lose the easy pounds quite quickly, especially if very overweight. Then slowly resistance sets in, weight loss slows down and one day the body resists a little more than on other days and weight loss comes to a halt. The dreaded high-risk stagnation plateau has been reached. The diet is followed just as carefully but the scales refuse to budge. The danger here is that motivation wavers, temptation rears its ugly head again, and small lapses fuel the stagnation. A large number of women 'in stagnation' give up, try again, chop and change and sooner or later abandon their diet altogether. It is extremely important to make sure there is no abnormal water retention, no hormonal imbalance or thyroid deficiency as these can put paid to the very best diet. If the results prove negative, the diet needs to be stepped up and certainly not toned down.

Now when the risk of giving up is high, the role that exercise plays becomes *crucial*. A body that has started to resist dieting cuts down its energy consumption and extracts every last calorie from its food intake, blocking weight loss long enough for the diet to fail. But if when the situation is blocked the forces present are in equilibrium, like the two sides of a pair of scales, and there is a sudden dose of 'prescribed exercise' this confuses the body, breaking the stalemate. Resistance gives way, the plateau collapses, the scales move, a victory is scored, weight drops, spirits rise, belief in the dieting programme is reinforced and the vicious circle becomes a virtuous one.

The truly determined will of course get their results by following the diet but the risks are high as it is difficult to foresee how long a stagnation phase may last. As a pre-emptive strike, I prescribe what I call a 'blitz operation' over a very brief period of time that dictates:

- Four days of the Attack diet's pure proteins without any deviation
- Restricting salt intake as much as possible
- Two litres of water with a low mineral content
- Getting to sleep as early as possible (sleep before midnight is much more beneficial than after)

- Adding a plant detox agent to drinks to eliminate any hidden water retention
- And, above all, WALKING FOR 60 MINUTES A DAY FOR FOUR DAYS

These six elements make up my anti-stagnation shock prescription and very often it is the walking that makes all the difference. So if one day you happen to encounter stagnation, don't forget what I have prescribed and be aware that while you are losing weight it is practically always inevitable that you'll go through a stagnation plateau. What counts is getting off it, and that is where exercise has a role to play.

Having observed on a daily basis how exceptionally effective exercise is when simple, but prescribed with firm guidance and precision, I decided to introduce this new 'PE' – Prescribed Exercise – front into the action plan and this book, which contains its essence.

It is more than 15 years since this book was first published, and today I am duty bound to record that this physical protocol is not a mere addition or marginal improvement; it is a transplant that radically changes the method's nature and results. My programme's two-pronged attack now offers no mercy for weight problems and weight stagnation.

Since I have been 'prescribing' exercise as a medicine with dosage and frequency and since I have been explaining and demonstrating its importance backed up by evidence – by comparing dieting on its own to dieting plus exercise – I have seen that even the most recalcitrant, lazy, busy people, and in particular those most resistant to dieting, totally believe in it, astonished by their results. What is more, they claim that they always knew, but did not truly believe it. Prescribing is vitally important because of this gap between knowing and believing.

I am asking you, therefore, to look upon exercise with different eyes, as a formidable weapon that has never before been properly deployed.

I can and must guarantee that if you follow my four-phase programme, from its Attack phase through to permanent stabilization, and my prescribed exercise programme, you will achieve your True Weight and you will maintain it, however resistant to dieting you are. Not only will you lose weight, you will be cured of being overweight.

PE – THE PRESCRIBED EXERCISE PROGRAMME IN DAILY PRACTICE

The reason why we are not properly encouraged to be active is that nobody believes in it, neither the doctors prescribing slimming treatments nor those following the treatments. Up until now, those prescribing have always been happy simply to recite politically correct common-sense advice such as: 'Try and be a bit more active, find time and make an effort.' Put like this, there is absolutely NO likelihood of such advice being followed, because whoever phrased it plainly did not really believe in it.

Nowadays, in many countries, over half the population is overweight. Faced with this progression, mankind faces a tendentious question. Should we allow our species to evolve and become overweight, a species turned adipose through overeating to compensate for the discordance of the world we now live in? Or should we say no to obesity and do we have the means to say no? My honest belief is that without consciously asking this question, society is choosing by default to tolerate widespread obesity. Of course you will hear ministers and high officials warn us about overeating and sedentary behaviour but nothing is actually being done to put a stop to it.

Since you are reading a book that sets out ways of tackling weight problems, you know my opinion. So my attempt to optimize my method will come as no surprise to you, a method to which I have devoted all my energy from the day my overweight publisher started me off on this journey. And I see in exercise the strategic element that, together with my diet, gives you what you need to make a personal choice about your body, your body image and whether you want to belong to the fat planet. If you really want to lose weight permanently as effectively as possible and with minimum frustration, you must follow my exercise instructions, which I have minimized and incorporated into the four phases of my programme.

The most frequently cited reason for only dieting and avoiding or getting round taking exercise is lack of time, which is a poor excuse. Experience proves that people who want to slim put themselves through beauty and body treatments that are infinitely more inconvenient and time-consuming than any exercise. Here again it all comes down to being totally convinced that exercise has a genuine role to play in losing weight, that it is definitely not just an add-on to a diet, but that together they form a coalition that doubles your chances of successfully shedding pounds in the short, medium and, even more so, the long term.

The Main Player: Walking

Of all human activities walking is the most natural

For anthropologists, man stopped being a great ape when he stood up on his two lower limbs and walked. After this decisive moment, all his activities, how he moved, how he hunted and protected himself, changed forever. His hands were freed up to interact with his brain, which could undertake more complex tasks, opening the way for intelligence, consciousness, language and culture. This tells us how deeply walking is ingrained and woven into the original structure of our brains and first behaviour patterns.

In our stressful and unnatural environment, walking has turned into both a waste of time and a loss of earnings for those who manufacture ways of transporting us, and in the current economic climate is an activity to be avoided and belittled. Why walk when we have escalators, lifts, bikes, mopeds, cars and electric scooters?

I have deliberately chosen walking to be my firm ally in the fight against weight problems as it is part and parcel of our humanity, a true celebration of our origins, inscribed in our nature and genes. Walking is one of the best ways of fighting against the artificiality of our way of life. It forces us to remain human, to use our bodies to move around, and it rewards us by secreting endorphins, the pleasure they provide proving that our body is satisfied. By walking we do ourselves good; as we gradually find pleasure in it, we end up needing to walk.

Walking is the simplest of all physical activities

As an embryo, each human baby reproduces a speeded-up version of the animal kingdom's long evolution from fish to mammal then ape. When a human baby is born, it continues with its programming; it learns to stand up and then to walk. As it takes its first steps it seems to be saying to its parents, 'I am one of your kind.' From this moment on, man walks as he breathes, as if this were the most natural thing in the world. Indeed, walking is so simple and automatic that it allows you to do almost anything else at the same time. When you are out walking you can think, plan your day, talk to your fellow walker or make a phone call. Life does not come to a halt when you are out walking.

Walking is the least tiring exercise and feasible for almost everyone

You can walk for hours without getting tired. The physical effort is spread widely over areas of bones and muscles. For a serious hike you need proper walking shoes but normal shoes, even ladies' heels, are fine for everyday walking to lose weight. Walking does not make you sweat unduly and you can walk whenever there is an opportunity, wearing whatever you want. There is no need for any sports gear, showering or change of clothes.

Walking exercises the greatest number of muscles at the same time

It is hard to imagine the complexity of what is such a simple and spontaneous activity. Huge investment has been required for cyberneticists to analyze and reproduce walking with science-fiction robots or to help those with motor disability. What is more, the muscles most involved in walking are the body's biggest 'load-bearers', i.e. they burn up the most calories. The muscles most involved are:

- The quadriceps. At the front of the thighs, they are by far the body's biggest muscles. They raise and push forwards the thigh and leg.
- The hamstrings, which form the back of the thigh and move your leg backwards.
- The buttock muscles. Very powerful and bulky, their job is to complete the backwards movement of the step. When these muscle masses sag, this shows that they are not being used enough for their primary function, which is walking.

- The stomach muscles, which actively contribute to walking as they contract with each step forwards.
- The calf muscles, smaller and more slender, but some of the most heavily used when you take a step.

Secondary muscles that also contribute:

- The pelvis's stabilizing muscles. They form a muscular crown surrounding the pelvis which prevents it from collapsing when the body is standing up. External abductors, internal adductors, abdominal muscles at the front and spinal muscles at the back.
- The symmetrical tibialis anterior muscles in front of the calf muscles. They raise the foot up so that it does not flatten or scrape the ground as you take a stride. Walking greatly develops these muscles.
- The arm and shoulder muscles which contribute less than the others but they can be used a great deal in power walking, such as Nordic walking.

That we use all these muscles, many of them fuel guzzlers, and at the same time, explains why so many calories get burnt.

Walking is the exercise that most helps you slim
This may come as a surprise but walking burns up as many calories as playing tennis and many other sports. Calorie-burning is optimized because it is a constant and uninterrupted activity whereas in a tennis match half your

time is spent with breaks in play and waiting for the ball to return. Optimized calorie-burning is also down to the fact that walking is totally bound up with daily life and can be undertaken at a moment's notice to fill in some spare time, anywhere and at any hour of the day or night.

In permanent stabilization walking is the most useful exercise

If it proves its worth when you are losing weight it is the only activity that can be accepted as part of your core of new habits, to be kept firstly through the Consolidation phase but so much more usefully in the long term throughout permanent stabilization, which is such a crucial period. For all the reasons previously mentioned – easy, natural, healthy and free from danger – walking is the activity that we will most easily agree to undertake regularly.

For obese people walking is the only risk-free exercise

And this is with results and effectiveness proportionate to the excess weight they are carrying around with them; and, above all, without danger of injury or cardiovascular risk. Never forget that an obese or even an overweight person is carrying a load. Carrying an extra 30 pounds may be looked upon in its own right as a sport but only if it is moved around through walking. Quite the reverse happens with, say, swimming or cycling when the weight is not being carried and the activity takes place more or less under weightless conditions. The heavier you are the better it is to walk.

Finally, walking is the exercise that best protects against ageing

Walking is the best way to keep the body's main functions going: circulation, respiration, bones, hormones, muscles and mental wellbeing. These are not so well cared for if we do not walk, so we age more quickly. Walking for 30 minutes a day, as well as helping us lose weight and stabilize it, allows us to live longer and in better physical condition. Walking is also bound up with mental health. For the physical effort required it is the activity that gets the brain secreting the most chemical mediators. It secretes endorphins, the cerebral mediators for pleasure, and serotonin, the 'happiness hormone'. Serotonin deficiency contributes to the onset of depression.

How to Walk During the Diet's Four Phases

From reading the previous pages you will have understood why I encourage you to walk and embrace this natural activity. As part of my programme, walking is to be combined with the diet based on the special features and purpose of each of its phases.

In the Attack phase, 20 minutes a day.
In the Cruise phase, 30 minutes a day.
If stagnation lasts longer than seven days, increase
    this to 60 minutes a day for four days.
In the Consolidation phase, 25 minutes a day.
In the permanent Stabilization phase, you must
    absolutely stick to 20 minutes a day.

- In the Attack phase, which lasts two to seven days, or even ten days in certain cases, walking is practically the only exercise prescribed capable of maximizing results without producing fatigue and an increased appetite. The aim is to set off like a shot and achieve a weight loss so dazzling it bolsters motivation. As you are making this effort, I prescribe 20 minutes' walking per day. Unless you already have particular habits and affinities, any more or less is not recommended.

  In general, with two days of pure proteins you lose between 1lb 12oz and 2lb 4oz, or 2lb 11oz if you add walking. For obese people, especially if their hips, knees and ankles are fragile, I recommend splitting the walking into two ten-minute doses.

- In the Cruise phase, the aim is to continue losing weight come hell or high water. Surprised by the attack your body is now trying to regain control and resist. To counter this risk, I prescribe a 30-minute dose of walking per day. Walking is particularly crucial in this phase. It may well be cold outside, it may well seem that you have no time, but just do it and go and walk; I guarantee you that the expected benefits will far outstrip what you may imagine. During this phase, despite the diet, your body will inevitably slam on the brakes and succeed in slowing down and then putting a stop to your weight loss. When stagnation is unmerited and unexplained, and no cause can be identified such as high water retention, thyroid deficiency, hormonal imbalance or use of weight gain-inducing medicine (cortisone, anti-depressants), it is advisable to increase walking from 30 to 60 minutes a day for four days. This can be split into two 30-minute periods.

- In the Consolidation phase, the aim is to make the transition from total dieting to non-dieting. Some look forward to this moment, but most dread the diet opening up to allow in new foods, which they fear will overturn their achievements. It always surprises me when men and women who were once great or chaotic eaters ask me why they have to leave the straight and narrow path of proteins and vegetables; the way is limited but clearly marked out, completely reassuring and not beset with temptation. My answer is because they need to eat spontaneously again and have an adult relationship with food.

  In Consolidation I prescribe a non-negotiable 25-minute dose of walking per day.

  This is a very important period at the end of which you will not only have achieved but also consolidated your weight.

- In the permanent Stabilization phase, the aim is to return to normal life and never put on a pound again. This 'never again' dictates a minimum but permanent prescription. The word 'permanent' is, of course, worrying but I guarantee you that anyone who tries to ignore the fact that they are prone to being overweight will soon put those shed pounds back on. You must be determined to protect your new weight and see the fully deployed Consolidation diet as a safe base, a set of pointers that make up a healthy, frugal but extremely safe diet. From this base, except for your safety rampart, the three measures, you can choose anything. You know them but it never harms to be reminded of the essentials: protein Thursdays, giving up lifts and escalators, and three tablespoons of oat bran.

In this phase, which I consider to be the most important BY FAR, I prescribe a 20-minute dose of walking per day. It is not much, not much at all, the borderline for what makes our bodies intrinsically human.

The Best Way to Walk

Walking, combined with my diet and to optimize its results, is neither specialized like Nordic walking nor is it just like walking round the shops. This is brisk walking: imagine you have to get to the post office before going to work and you have no time to lose. Nothing more, nothing less. You can also enhance your walking by choosing the best time of day and by adding some specific extras.

Walking to digest

Walking straight after a meal increases calorie combustion by 30 per cent. If within 30 minutes of finishing a meal you get up and walk, not only will you burn up what is required for the walking but at the same time you will raise the thermal effect of digestion and your body heat which effectively lowers the meal's caloric value by as much. Whether festive or naughty, the more copious your meal, the more calories you will have consumed. So here you have a way, albeit small, of repairing possible misdemeanours while dieting.

Best foot backwards

This is not about walking backwards but making full use of the moment when one leg is behind, to increase calorie-combustion and tone 'forgotten' muscles.

Seasoned walkers look straight ahead as they walk, instinctively searching in front of them for foothold, which is called the forward walking time. The front foot is in the air, the thigh is following while the other leg passively goes into a backward position. The forward movement time sets the quadriceps to work. The abdominal muscles are also made to work, as is the hamstring connected to the tibia, which with each step lifts up before the foot to stop it from scuffing the ground.

To walk better, you also need to work the muscles controlling the back leg. Once the foot has finished taking the forward step, it returns to the vertical position and passively starts to take up the position of back leg; here you take control and turn this into an active time. Instead of letting your foot go back like a pendulum, keep it on the ground momentarily by contracting your buttock muscle and the hamstring. Doing this burns twice the calories and makes the back of your body work as hard as the front.

Walking tall

Beneficial at any age, this is a marvellous way of getting more out of your walking. We are not talking about an exercise here but how you go about your life. What exactly do we mean by standing up straight? Quite simply, aligning your head with your chest, elongating your neck and drawing your shoulders backwards and downwards.

For young people, adopting this posture gives them natural elegance, grace and style. It goes without saying that such rare attributes are eminently seductive and instil a feeling of self-worth. This is even before we consider the calories consumed by standing up straight if you are not used to it, because this position gets an impressive number of different muscles working.

For a man or woman aged over 50, standing upright and even more so walking with their head held high makes them look younger. How is this so? As a simple experiment, look around you. After wrinkles, greying hair and a sagging jaw line, one of the first signs of ageing is stooping forwards with a scrunched-up neck. To my mind, stooping ages you far more than being overweight. So lose weight by following the diet and walking tall!

FOUR KEY EXERCISES FOR FOUR KEY AREAS

Many dieters with a sedentary lifestyle look for magical ways of speeding up their physical exercise, but they are swamped by a never-ending array of different exercises and become paralyzed by the sheer number, unable to choose. During my time as a practitioner dealing with weight problems, I have developed an ability to take control and a preference for supervising my patients directly. Not out of a taste for authority – without question I prefer helping and being on the same emotional wavelength

– but because I am convinced that instructions that are simple, concrete, reliable, unambiguous and firm make monitoring and following these instructions much easier. So I have chosen four exercises that address two concerns: weight loss in the most muscular areas and intensity of calorie combustion. This is also in response to requests from patients whose weight loss has resulted in flabbiness and 'surplus skin' in the four most vulnerable areas: the stomach, arms, buttocks and thighs.

A Body Losing Weight Has Four Vulnerable Areas

After losing over 15 pounds a race develops between the disappearing fat and the retracting skin. In fact, fat disappears quicker than the skin is able to retract, and this disparity is even more notable in areas where the skin is very fine and most put to use.

Women, therefore, complain most commonly about surplus skin and loss of elasticity in these four areas:

- A wobbly, potbellied stomach. When you slim, the loss of weight and adipose tissue affects the exterior just as much as the interior, the layer of fat around the stomach muscles just as much as the internal fat surrounding the intestines. When the internal fat melts away, this makes the muscles less tense and the stomach appears wobbly and sticks out. When the external fat disappears the skin now becomes less firm. After weight loss the skin retracts, but so slowly that it takes six months for it to reach its best tonicity. After six months you cannot hope for any further improvement but you should not attempt anything radical beforehand. As for the stomach's potbellied appearance, this is due to the muscle wall relaxing. To tone it and have a flat stomach again you have to work the abdominal muscles with traditional abdominal exercises. There are a very large number of these, too many for the uninitiated. I have devised my own and suggest only one as this is enough but it must be done every day without fail.

- The back of the arms. It is mostly those women who had thick arms before slimming who complain about them turning flabby. After losing weight, the arms are not so large but the skin has not shrunk enough so the back of the arm hangs down. Here again I use a single exercise so that the instructions remain clear and simple.

- Drooping, sagging buttocks. Women's buttocks are naturally divided between large load-bearing muscles and a thick cushion of fat that makes sitting more comfortable and highlights their sexuality. A sedentary woman's buttock muscles show signs of atrophy and as soon as she sheds pounds she quickly loses her adipose cushion leaving her with soft, sagging buttocks and much reduced sex appeal. For this very common occurrence I use one complete, single but satisfactory exercise.

- Flabby thighs. This mostly affects gynoid type women who put on weight in the lower body: hips, thighs and knees. With substantial weight loss the slimmed thighs are less firm and their skin covering is much less stretched. Again I prescribe a single exercise that can develop the quadriceps and completely tone up the thighs, restoring their curves.

1. The Dukan Diet Special

This exercise is my Swiss army knife. I devised it for myself and have been using it for more than 20 years. Apart from walking, if there is only one exercise you ever stick to I would ask you to choose this one. Why? Because it is simple and can be incorporated effortlessly into your daily routine. Short and sweet, you do it in bed, once when you wake up and again before you go to sleep. It is exceptionally effective and enables you to work a large range of muscle groups – stomach, thigh and arm.

Position a pillow and a cushion on your bed to make a comfortable inclined plane. Lie down with your back on this inclined plane. Bend your knees and with your arms outstretched hold your knees however is best for you, either clasping them from above or on the inside or outside. In this half-supine position, raise your chest vertically using only your stomach muscles and without any help from your arms. Then lower yourself on to your cushion and pillow support. Try to do this 15 times without using your arms.

Once you have managed this 15 times, start again from scratch, lifting yourself up with your arm muscles now instead of your stomach muscles. Raise your chest to a vertical position, pulling only with your biceps which are much weaker than your stomach muscles. Try to do this

15 times, which makes 30 times in total for your morning session.

In the evening, when you lie down to sleep, follow the same sequence, bringing the total to 60 times so that from day one you are building up firmness in your abdominal wall and biceps. This double exercise, which also works your thigh muscles, takes only a minute or so both morning and evening.

Every day try to add one more to both the stomach and arm muscles exercises, both morning and evening, i.e. 31 + 31 on the second day, 32 + 32 on the third day, and 36 + 36 by the end of the first week. The goal is to reach 70 + 70 by the end of the first month and in time to manage 100 in the morning and another 100 in the evening. By the time you manage this, these 200 exercises will only take you three minutes which is hardly anything.

Thanks to this incredibly effective but non-time-consuming exercise, your once flabby and potbellied stomach will become toned and flat again.

2. The Buttock Muscles Special

This is another exercise I do every day immediately after the first one while still in bed when I wake up and before I go to sleep. It is extremely effective: the buttocks, back of the arms and thighs warm up very quickly, very powerfully, and I feel them getting toned. Moreover, to my mind this exercise is fun for, as you will see, it has a 'trampoline' element.

Start by removing the pillow and cushion – you do this exercise lying flat. Lie on your back with your arms outstretched on the bed. Bring your knees up to your thighs to form a right angle. In this position, pushing down both on your outstretched arms and also on your feet and the muscles in the back of the thighs, make a bridge shape by raising your buttocks towards the ceiling until your chest and legs are aligned on a perfectly sloping straight line. Once you are aligned, lower yourself quickly, bounce off the mattress and go up again until you form a straight line again. The trampoline effect makes the exercise easier and helps you keep going until you feel warmth and tone creeping into the back of your arms, thighs and in your buttocks. This is a major exercise.

Again, start off doing it 30 times and then another 30 times later when you go to bed. 60 times a day will not take more than a minute and a half as you do one after the other. If you cannot manage 30 times, this means your pelvis and backside are very heavy and your muscle base in particular is weak or atrophied. If this is so, do not worry; do a little less knowing that these muscles quickly adapt and that before long you will manage it. However, try to do a minimum of ten lifts in the morning and then again in the evening, because your difficulties prove that you really need to do this exercise.

Then as with the previous exercise, try and add another one each day so that eventually you do 100 in the morning and 100 at night. By then your chest and pelvis will look slimmer from the weight loss, and toned and muscular through combining these two exceptional exercises.

3. The Thighs Special

This exercise has a double benefit: it uses up the most calories as it works the body's biggest muscle, the quadriceps, which as its name suggests is made up of four muscle sheaths. It also tackles one of the areas most affected by cellulite, where weight loss and the flabbiness this causes can make the cellulite soft, which is its worst fate.

This exercise aims to burn up calories and at the same time fill the empty space where the fat used to be with firm thigh muscle. It is one of the simplest and most effective and therefore satisfies my quest for a single exercise.

Stand, if possible in front of a mirror, placing your feet slightly apart so that you are firm and steady and support yourself by placing both hands on a table or sink. Slowly crouch down, bending your knees until your buttocks touch your heels. Then straighten up and return to your starting position.

Although difficult this exercise produces great results. By definition how well it goes depends on your weight, where this weight is concentrated and how fit you are. If you are very stout – over 15 stone – you will have trouble doing it once. If this is so, try the exercise without going the whole way; do what you can and as you progress you can test your weight loss and how it impacts on your physical performance. As the days and weeks pass, and through practice, the time will come when you can complete your first whole exercise. Soon afterwards you will do a second and then you will be away and achieving the ideal number for someone who is overweight, a sequence of 15, which means you are not far off your True Weight.

If from the very first day you can manage this exercise at least once, you can get up to 15 in two weeks by adding another one each day as long as you feel able and by not allowing yourself to go into reverse, unless it is to let your muscles recover a little by going back to what you did the day before. As soon as you have finished your first sequence of 15, aim for 30 but take your time, another one every week suits me fine. Once you have got to 30 you will have firm, nicely curved thighs and eight little monster muscles, four per quadriceps, which will spend their time burning up calories day and night. Because the good news about your muscles is that they continue to burn calories *after you have finished exercising*. Although at a lower rate than during exercise, calorie combustion carries on continually day and night for 72 hours and then it stops. This is why it is important to keep going and link the exercises to each other; ideally you should be active every single day.

4. The Flabby Arms Special

Women's arms provide a good indication of their weight problem history, the thickness and quality of their skin and their morphology type. Most women with cellulite on their thighs also have thick arms. When these women lose weight they lose it more easily from their arms than from their thighs and very often the result is flabby skin. There are not many solutions for this common problem. Creams do not work; surgery is not advised as it leaves too much scarring. This is my favourite exercise for the arms: it is comprehensive, simple and effective, and the only one you need.

The advantage of this exercise is that it works two opposing muscles simultaneously, the biceps in the front of the arm and the triceps in the back, so that it develops the muscles throughout the fleshy area, tautening the flabby skin integument and helping when the flabbiness is not too obvious as well as when it is.

Stand up and hold a one and a half litre bottle of water, or object of similar weight. Start the exercise with your arms by your side, stretching down towards the ground. Then bend your forearm, bringing the bottle up to touch your shoulder. Stretch your arm and bring it back down to the original vertical position, then take it further behind you with your arm stretched back as far as possible until you reach a horizontal position or even further. The first part of this exercise contracts the biceps, the second the triceps and together they tone and increase the arm's muscle mass, tautening the covering skin.

The complete exercise should be done 15 times, for each arm, to increase the muscle mass sufficiently so that the skin is tensed. Try and do as much as you can and if you can keep it up then go for it as a muscle only undergoes hypertrophy when under maximum pressure. Once you have done this exercise 15 times a day for a week, try to increase each week first to 20 then to 25 so that by the end of the first month you can manage 30 in succession. After that be guided by how you feel but already your arms will be firmer and more muscular.

Remember too that skin that has become slack after slimming needs six months to completely finish retracting. After this time do not expect any spontaneous improvement. So the watchword for these four exercises is: build up the muscles, tighten your skin from within and wait for it to fully retract.

By enabling you to lose more weight, more quickly, and to feel better, more toned and lovely, exercise helps you achieve a personal project and OBTAIN SUCCESS. And you must be aware that success is one of the main sources of self-fulfilment and self-realization, one of the pleasures and rewards most bound up with self-esteem, fulfilment and happiness.

HOW TO BENEFIT MOST FROM MY DIET WHILE AVOIDING RISKS

Please always bear in mind that being overweight, obese or having diabetes from being overweight is directly responsible for over 50,000 deaths in France each year. When people talk about the side effects of a slimming method, this should always be seen in the context of its primary advantage, which is to keep the individual alive.

I created this method more than 35 years ago. For more than ten years now it has been shared and used in 30 or so countries and has spontaneously forged a community of 10–15 million people across the world. During this time when my method has been used by so many people, I have received a great number of messages with thanks and success stories of both the short as well as the medium and long term. On the other hand, in over 40 years I've never been told about any sort of setback, any difficulty or harmfulness or received a single complaint from a user. Yes, there are minor secondary effects, but never any primary ones.

However, since my method is being used ever more widely, and a growing number of overweight individuals are continuing and will continue to make it their own, and since I can no longer always be there to answer their questions, I would like to make sure that no one makes any mistakes when interpreting my instructions.

Talk to Your GP

The first recommendation I'd make to any reader about to start my diet with the intention of losing well over a stone is to inform your GP. Better still, ask for their support. Even better, ask for their help.

How?

If you have a good GP, they are bound to be snowed under, with no time to spare. So perhaps they won't manage to look after your weight loss programme themselves, but they can monitor you medically. Your doctor knows you and so is the person best placed to realize if there is anything in your medical history to counter-indicate losing weight. And your doctor can also advise you against trying to lose weight if you don't actually need to because your weight is medically 'normal'. If your doctor agrees to supervise you as you follow my method, it would be ideal if they started by prescribing routine blood tests. What should you be looking for? Dyslipidaemia (excess cholesterol, good HDL and bad LDL levels or excess triglycerides), as with a case of diabetes or pre-diabetes, so you can have the pleasure of watching these levels drop, which is what practically always happens when fat and sugar intake is reduced.

Whenever someone starts a high protein diet, it is

useful to check that there is no nascent or established kidney failure. What is kidney failure? This is when a kidney is lazy, tired or diseased. To get a very accurate idea of how well your kidneys are working, the blood tests prescribed need only include results for creatinine, the speed with which it is eliminated and the level of urea. With very severe kidney failure, diets must be avoided where the kidneys have to eliminate waste from proteins. If the kidneys are simply tired, all you need do is drink one and a half litres of water, avoid salty foods, alcohol and any medication that is harsh for the kidneys so as not to tire them any further. And if the kidneys are simply lazy, then all you need to do is drink. Finally, by taking these simple blood tests you can also see how well your thyroid is working, and whether you have a lazy thyroid or thyroid insufficiency. The test will check the level of three hormones: TSH, T4 and T3. If you get this done when you start on the diet, you can avoid coming up against a body that will simply refuse to lose weight and will resist any diet, even the most effective ones. These tests are what I have always prescribed beforehand to my personal patients and I strongly recommend them to my readers too. If any major biological imbalance is discovered, then medical supervision becomes a must; and becoming aware of a problem strengthens the individual's resolve to rebalance these disorders.

How to Manage Any Vulnerability You May Have as You Embark on My Diet

If you are overweight, and especially if you have been carrying a lot of extra weight over a long period and you are over 45, it is highly likely that you will display small signs of fragility, clinical or biological manifestations linked to excessive eating and being overweight. Losing this well-established and often resistant weight will therefore need to be spread out over time. That being the case, how can you slim down with the best chance of improving these clinical or simply biological signs of excess, or even be rid of them altogether? How do you avoid any risk of nutritional deficiency? And finally, how do you avoid or alleviate any unwanted outcomes or side effects from the diet?

- If you are vulnerable to lipids and predisposed to cholesterol or if you are simply worried about their onset, then take great care not to mix up lean and fatty meats. Please try to remember that in my method you are not allowed pork or lamb, and that veal and beef are permitted so long as you avoid rib steak and chops as these are too marbled with fat.

  What's more, although you are allowed to eat these meats without any restriction, as far as you are concerned I would ask that you always opt for fish, and in particular for oily fish such as salmon, sardines, mackerel and tuna whose fats 'work to clear' the arteries. Land animal fat blocks the vessels a little, while fat from sea creatures will clear them. Also, you may eat the white part of any shellfish, but make sure you avoid the coral wherever it is: scallop lobes, on prawn heads etc.

Furthermore, if you have excessive cholesterol, remember to remove the skin from your poultry, avoid offal and eat no more than three or four egg yolks a week – but you may have as much egg white as you wish: American-style egg white omelettes or, if you are really hungry, use a single yolk with two, three or four whites. Armed with these precautionary measures, you stand a good chance of improving your levels.

- If you are vulnerable to sugar, i.e. you simply have a genetic predisposition to diabetes, onset diabetes or even well-established diabetes, you have EVERYTHING to gain from slimming down – but you will need to stick to a few rules.

– If you have type 1 diabetes

i.e. you use insulin, you will be supervised not only by your GP but also by a diabetes specialist. As far as you are concerned, the risk is not of hyperglycaemia but of brief episodes of hypoglycaemia, which can cause serious discomfort. My diet may be very good for you, but only on the express condition that your diabetes specialist takes complete charge so that your weight loss programme fits around your insulin requirements. The best way of making sure that the weight-loss diet is safe for an insulin dependent diabetic is to ensure that it includes three oat bran galettes a day: one in the morning at breakfast, one at lunchtime and one in the evening. Oat bran slows down the absorption of sugars and too fast-acting carbohydrates, thereby avoiding insulin peaks, which bring on hypoglycaemia. You won't be cured, but you'll need less insulin, i.e. you'll be healthier.

– If you have type 2 diabetes

i.e. instead of insulin you use oral diabetes medicine – you'll be quite comfortable with my method, which combines losing weight with taking exercise. Nevertheless, it is crucial that you talk to your doctor about it because diabetes is a disorder that must absolutely be kept under control. So as far as you are concerned, you should stick with fish, alternate pure protein days with protein and vegetables and eat two oat bran galettes a day: one in the morning and one in the evening for pleasure, so that you feel full and to help you control your diabetes.

In your case, your early morning glycaemia will reduce in no time at all. If you have a blood glucose meter, you'll notice the change from the first week.

– If you just have pre-diabetes, if you developed gestational diabetes during one or more pregnancies or if diabetes simply runs in your family, i.e. a direct relative has it or has had it – my method has been devised for you. Talk to your doctor about the programme and follow it as closely as possible since you may quite simply 'be cured', and manage to get off the path that might be leading you there.

• If you have a weak kidney, it is important that you are

aware of this. What exactly does having a weak kidney mean? The kidney is the organ that works to purify the body by constantly filtering our blood to get rid of waste products. As is the case with any organ, some kidneys are better genetically at doing their job than others. Some kidneys have been weakened by illness, kidney stones, infections and, lastly, female kidneys may work less effectively because of pregnancies, the pre-menopause, water retention and oversensitivity to ovarian hormones. There are also serious diseases that prevent the kidneys from working properly: kidney failure.

If you suffer from serious kidney failure that might involve having to undergo regular dialysis, it is clear that dieting under such circumstances is not advised, whatever the diet, and especially not high-protein ones since metabolizing such diets releases waste products, which the kidneys would struggle to eliminate. Such cases have generally already been clearly identified and are being monitored in hospital.

If a person is extremely overweight or dangerously obese, they need to be medically supervised and a kidney specialist must take all the decisions and take charge of the treatment. I very strongly advise against any person with kidney failure following my diet on their own.

– There may be less serious renal failure, which does not present clinical signs but which shows up on biological testing and renal function markers such as urea, creatinine and kidney filtration rates. Whenever these markers are failing, this is when your doctor plays a particularly useful role as they will know whether any increase in these markers should be taken seriously or not, and they can track any developments through repeated testing. Only your doctor is in a position to determine whether the dangers from being overweight outweigh those of accumulating waste products.

– Finally, some kidneys are lazy or have poor drainage and this laziness only manifests itself through a strong tendency to retain water in body tissue. In such cases, it is important to drink enough to help the kidneys filter, but without exceeding one and a half litres so as to avoid running the risk of retaining this water. It is also important to cut back on salt and any other food with a high waste component such as deli meats, tinned and ready-cooked food and alcohol. For anyone with a lazy kidney, it is again vital that you ask your doctor for their opinion as they will need to check your kidney function and monitor you for any fluctuations for as long as you follow the diet.

Dieting and Deficiencies

Any weight-loss diet, whatever it is, may if it is not followed correctly or is too restrictive result in insufficient micronutrient intake, leading to deficits and, in certain extreme cases, to deficiency. However, we need to remind ourselves that nowadays such deficiencies are extremely rare. The first vitamin, vitamin C, was discovered when sailors went away on long trips and were without fresh vegetables for over six months, then started eating green vegetables again. Since working as a nutritionist, I've come across vitamin deficits, but never a genuine deficiency.

As you know, my programme starts with an Attack phase based on exclusively eating 72 lean protein foods. Usually this phase lasts two to seven days depending on how many pounds there are to lose, i.e. four days on average for someone who wants to lose one and a half stone. In four days, there is ABSOLUTELY NO risk of any deficit, even the slightest, and even less of any deficiency.

Twenty-eight vegetables get added with the Cruise phase and are eaten on alternate days until you achieve your True Weight.

Let's look at possible deficits during these first two phases, which concentrate on weight loss. Once you get to the third Consolidation phase, all food categories are included so there is no question then of any deficit.

- The first deficiency to fear with a weight-loss diet is lack of protein. There are some fashionable diets, such as the Lemon Diet, the Cabbage Soup Diet and the Beverly Hills with nothing but exotic fruit. Since the human body cannot synthesize proteins and needs them every eight hours, by the ninth hour it reacts immediately by taking them from your muscles or skin. The result is muscle loss, lack-lustre skin, hair and nails and less bone mineralization, which increases the risk of osteoporosis. My programme is probably the one with the least risk of any such deficiency as you can eat proteins 'as much as you like'. Of all the diets available, it offers you the best chance of preserving your muscle age.

- As far as vitamins are concerned, they fall into two categories. There are liposoluble vitamins, which are absorbed into the body through fatty tissue: including vitamins A, D and E. And then there are those that are soluble in water and mostly come from fruit and vegetables: hydrosoluble vitamins. By choosing carefully from the 100 authorised foods it is relatively easy to avoid any vitamin shortage.

– Vitamin A

This vitamin is mostly provided by calves' or chicken liver, eggs or oily fish, such as sardines, salmon, tuna and mackerel. However, intake comes mainly from its precursor, beta-carotene, found in abundance in certain vegetables that you can eat as much as you like of in my diet: spinach, parsley, carrots, green beans and chicory. So it would be difficult not to get enough vitamin A with my diet.

– Vitamin D

This vitamin is mostly synthesised in our skin when we are exposed to the sun. Apart from the traditional doses of cod liver oil, which people don't take nowadays, the best food source is simply salmon, the food most widely consumed by most of my patients and readers, followed by sardines, egg, herring and then far behind them mushrooms. In winter, a large section of the population lacks vitamin D. You'll notice this in the dosage that your doctor will have advised, and in this case it is a good idea to take supplements.

– Vitamin E

This vitamin is fat-soluble and is found particularly in oils, but also in cereal fibre. During the first two Attack and Cruise phases, you'll find it in oat bran, cocoa (also in fat-reduced cocoa), eggs, liver, meat, poultry and especially in oily fish.

– Vitamin B group

Apart from vitamin B12, the vitamins in this group are found more or less in all my diet's 100 foods, in oat bran in particular, but also in very large quantities in brewer's yeast, which I recommend you to take throughout your life. As for vitamin B12, it's a vitamin that is both rare and vital as a lack of it can lead to severe anaemia, which happens very frequently with women who have difficulty assimilating iron. There is no risk of this with my diet as it offers plenty of vitamin B12 and iron, both being found essentially in foods of animal origin: meat, poultry and fish. Vegetarians will find vitamin B12 in eggs and dairy products, but in far lesser quantities, however pure vegans who do not allow themselves to eat eggs or dairy produce must agree to take a supplement to avoid vitamin B12 deficit or deficiency, which can turn out to be quite dreadful.

– Vitamin C

This vitamin is thought to be found exclusively in fruit, which does not feature in the first two phases. However, this is not correct: it is found in virtually every vegetable, to be sure mostly in smaller amounts for most vegetables, but some have a far higher content than the average fruit. This is true for sweet peppers and cabbage (twice as much as in oranges) and in lesser concentration in tomatoes and green beans. However, as far as vitamin C content goes, the champion is parsley, which is up there on the podium close to kiwi fruit.

- Risk of micronutrient deficit.
  - Iron

Women are very often deficient in this micronutrient, especially when periods are too heavy or come too close together. There is no risk of any such shortage with my diet, as it is packed with foods of animal origin such as meat, poultry and fish, which are the best sources of iron.

- Selenium

Selenium is also found in products of animal origin, meat, fish, poultry, seafood and most especially oysters, which occupy prime position with the highest content.

- Zinc

Zinc is fairly well represented in products of animal origin, meat, milk and eggs; however, the overall champions are still oysters and common shellfish.

- The problem with salt. Regardless of diets, the French consume two to three times the recommended quantity of salt. In my diet, I advise against eating too much salt. Among the 100 foods in my two Attack and Cruise phases, only smoked salmon, lean hams and air-dried/wind-dried beef are industrially produced with added salt. Anyone prone to high blood pressure is advised to opt instead for marinated salmon and to cut down on air-dried/wind-dried beef – and if possible, buy it sliced at the counter rather than pre-packaged.

- Dietary fibre in the Dukan Diet. With the refining of flours and less interest in high-fibre foodstuffs, the consumption of dietary fibre has decreased considerably over the past century. In France, average dietary fibre intake has dropped from over 30g (1oz) per day to 15–20g (½oz). Nine out of ten French people do not eat enough dietary fibre.

During my diet's actual weight-loss period – Attack + Cruise – only the vegetables provide dietary fibre intake, which is not enough. However, this is rectified by eating oat bran, which is extremely high in fibre.

To conclude this overview of any possible risk of deficiency during my diet, it is obvious that to avoid any micronutrient intake deficit, you should begin by eating as much as you want because once you drop below a minimum calorie intake, it is hard to avoid missing out on certain nutrients and vitamins. So we need once again to remind ourselves that in my diet there is no restriction on calorie intake and that seeking to reduce it to achieve better results is of only limited value. You should only resort to restricting calories during stagnation periods. For an obese person with a lot of weight to lose, the weight-loss phases will last longer and this may increase the risk of a deficit. In both cases, it is advisable to take a multivitamin complex alongside the diet until your True Weight is achieved as this will immediately de facto rule out any risk of deficit.

100 NATURAL FOODS
THAT KEEP YOU HEALTHY

Eat as much as you like

Very Protein-Rich Foods

Meat and offal

1. Beef steak
2. Fillet of beef
3. Sirloin steak
4. Roast beef
5. Rump steak
6. Tongue
7. Bresaola, air-dried/wind-dried beef
8. Veal escalope
9. Veal chop
10. Kidney
11. Calf's liver
12. Pre-cooked ham slices (without any fat or rind)
13. Pre-cooked chicken and turkey slices (without any fat or rind)
14. Fat-reduced bacon
15. Game (venison, pheasant, partridge, hare, grouse)
16. Rabbit/hare

Fish

17. Bass
18. Cod (fresh)
19. Crab/ocean sticks (surimi)
20. Dab/lemon sole
21. Dover sole
22. Grey mullet
23. Haddock
24. Hake
25. Halibut
26. Herring
27. Mackerel
28. Monkfish
29. Plaice
30. Pollock/Coley
31. Rainbow trout/salmon trout
32. Red mullet
33. Salmon
34. Smoked salmon
35. Sardines
36. Sea bream
37. Skate
38. Swordfish
39. Tuna
40. Turbot
41. Whiting
42. Fish roe (cod, salmon, herring, mullet)

Seafood

43. Calamari/squid
44. Clams
45. Cockles
46. Crab
47. Crawfish/crayfish
48. Dublin Bay prawns
49. Lobster
50. Mediterranean prawn/gambas
51. Mussels
52. Oysters
53. Prawns
54. Scallops
55. Shrimps
56. Whelks

Poultry

57. Chicken
58. Poussin
59. Chicken liver
60. Guinea fowl
61. Ostrich
62. Pigeon
63. Quail
64. Turkey

Eggs

65. Hen's eggs
66. Quail's eggs

Non-fat dairy products

67. Non-fat cottage cheese
68. Non-fat fromage frais
69. Non-fat Greek yoghurt
70. Non-fat quark/non-fat yoghurt (plain or flavoured with aspartame)
71. Skimmed milk

Vegetable Proteins

72. Tofu and Seitan

Vegetables

73. Artichoke (globe)
74. Asparagus
75. Aubergine
76. Beetroot
77. Broccoli/purple sprouting broccoli
78. Cabbage: white/red/Savoy/cauliflower/Chinese leaves/kohlrabi/kale/Brussels sprout (all types of cabbage)
79. Carrot
80. Celery/celeriac
81. Chicory

82. Courgette
83. Cucumber
84. Fennel
85. French beans/string beans/mangetout
86. Leek
87. Mushrooms
88. Onion
89. Palm hearts
90. Peppers (sweet)
91. Pumpkin/marrow/squash
92. Radish
93. Rhubarb
94. Salad leaves: all types of lettuce/rocket/watercress/ alfalfa/curly endive/sorrel
95. Soya beans
96. Spinach
97. Swede
98. Swiss chard
99. Tomatoes
100. Turnip

AFTERWORD

This final chapter is, in essence, the extra chapter I wrote for the French edition that came out in September 2008. I have included it so that this book also has up-to-date information about research and developments concerning my method, which have taken place since the work first appeared, in 2000.

For any author who believes that they have a message to share, I hope with all my heart that they too experience what happened with this book, my eighteenth. Within a few years it became a standard reference work on the subject of weight loss, forging its own path and filling me with pride and joy.

After a slow start it discovered its readers and won them over. A rare phenomenon then took place that neither I nor my publisher have understood as sales rocketed and reached levels rarely achieved by a French author: when 2007 drew to a close this book was immediately behind *Harry Potter* on Amazon France and ever since has been one of the top selling titles each year.

An Amazing Book

The book owes this success to the enthusiasm of users who have benefited from it and have then worked tirelessly to spread the word, going out of their way to talk about it on the internet. In the space of four years, over 200 sites, forums and blogs were set up by anonymous users and volunteers, mostly women, who without knowing me became genuine instructors in my method.

Not only did I receive the affectionate loyalty of those who successfully lost weight by following my programme, but I also came to enjoy the support of many French GPs.

At the same time, my method made its way into other countries and cultures. The rights to the book were acquired by Italian, Korean, Thai, Spanish, Brazilian, Polish and British publishers. As much as I understood the success in France for the method I had created and crafted for my patients and then for a wider book-reading public, the stir created through the press and forums in other cultures as diverse as Brazil and Korea took me by surprise.

After the book appeared in other countries I received many letters from journalists and doctors telling me how they liked the method and the successful results they had achieved by following it. They all told me that however French the method may have appeared at the outset it had not seemed foreign to them. The 100 foods that make up the two actual slimming phases all come from our wealth of human foods. The 72 protein foods and the 28 vegetables form the basis of food for man in step with nature, hunter of proteins and gatherer of vegetables. I do not know of a country in the world where these foods are not eaten.

Moreover, the mention of 'as much as you want'

responds to the way we function, which is instinctive and natural for any living being. When the need makes itself felt, it compels you to drink or eat until you no longer feel hungry or thirsty, i.e. until there is a return to a biological equilibrium. And this need is all the more demanding when it is coupled with a desire or compulsion of a psychological and emotional nature. It is calorie-counting and having to stop yourself when faced with tempting food that runs counter to nature; it can be done but it creates frustration.

The Bulgarian phenomenon

In the meantime what I named the 'Bulgarian phenomenon' happened. A Bulgarian publisher had acquired the rights to the work. Not having the money to promote it, the book apeared without any frills or fanfare. In the first year the earnings were poor; the publisher was on the verge of giving it up when, true to its usual way of getting itself known – word of mouth – the book started out on its Bulgarian career. Within a few months it had become the bestselling book in the country. A five-page special feature in Sofia's leading daily newspaper sparked everything off and there I was in the middle of an explosion that today I still cannot quite understand but which is one of the high points in my life. Bulgaria, one of the poorest countries in Europe, home to nine million people wild about my method! (Since 2008, Poland has actually outstripped this success – the book topped the bestseller chart for all categories.)

This anecdote aside, however breathtaking it may be, I then started thinking about how the method no longer belonged to me. It had actually overtaken me to become the property of all those who needed it to lose weight. I had been lucky enough to put it together but it now had to live its own life because it had a future before it.

A Quick Aside: My Final Word on Low-calorie Diets

Today, after more than 40 years of daily practice as a nutritionist treating excess weight and obesity, I am convinced that one of the reasons why the struggle against weight problems has failed throughout the world is that supporters of low-calorie diets insist on continuing to use them.

In theory, this is the most logical of diets but in practice it is one of the worst. Why is this so? Because it is based on a model that works against the mindset of people who put on weight. It seems as if exact calorie-counting only takes the cold logic of figures into account, ignoring anything to do with feelings, emotions, pleasure and the need to find sensory gratification, which are the basic reasons why we put on weight.

Low-calorie diets tell you that you eat too much, or too many things that are bad or too rich. This is true, but it does not explain *why* you do it. And they also say that you will put on weight because you swallow too many calories, so if you cut down the number, you will lose weight.

Everything, but in tiny quantities, so you spend your day counting, one food after the other, to make sure you do not go over the number of calories allocated, whether it be 1,800 or 600. Such orders are the exact opposite of what goes on inside the head of a man or woman prone to put on weight. If they were able to follow such orders or complicated calculations, an overweight or obese person would never have become overweight or obese in the first place. If some dieters do manage to do it, then this is because they are exceptionally motivated and for the time it takes to lose weight they are happy to change their identity and character.

But what happens if you manage to get down to the weight you want? Can you then ask someone who put on weight because they had always eaten without counting to suddenly turn into a calorie-counter? In my work as a practitioner I have almost always dealt with men and women whose relationship with food is 'all or nothing'. As far as weight is concerned, these wonderful people openly confess that they are capable of switching from the strictest diet to total bingeing, 'eating anything and everything'.

To defend this counter-productive diet, which goes against nature, its supporters brandish the word: BALANCE – eat a *balanced* diet. But if they were capable of eating a balanced diet, overweight people would never become overweight. In over 40 years, I have not met a single person who *wants* to become big, fat or obese. If a woman becomes obese, it is because she was unable to resist eating. Asking a woman like this to eat only 900 calories a day will simply add to her confusion and suffering.

Low-calorie diets have been around for over 65 years. Wherever they are taught they have failed, but the people who still use them do not want to acknowledge their failure. Moreover, by definition, the recommendation to cut down and count calories makes any hope of stabilizing the weight achieved impossible. The only exception is the Weight Watchers method. Through its points system, it prescribes food-counting but it is not the diet itself that is innovative and effective; it is their meetings, which at the time were a real revolution. Weight Watchers are, to my mind, the only ones who can claim to have slowed down the increase in weight problems in the world.

However, low-calorie diets without any real monitoring are almost automatically doomed to failure. Besides, just like powder sachet diets but for different reasons, they are dying out because nowadays users can swap information and pass on their own experiences via websites, forums, blogs and Twitter. And I hope that it will be pressure from the very people who actually follow diets that will bring about the end of these diets from a bygone era.

ABOUT THE AUTHOR

Pierre Dukan has specialized in human nutrition since 1973. He is the author of many works on nutrition, scientific works as well as those for the general public, and regularly writes in the press and appears on television.

The popularity of Dukan's methods and works in countries as different in culture as Korea or Bulgaria show how he has become the most widely read French nutritionist in the world. In 2009, the *Dukan Method* was the best-selling book in Poland.

In 1975, Dukan saw that the strategies being adopted to tackle the surge in weight problems and the repercussions on health were not working. In June 1976, he wrote in a scientific journal: 'We are confronted daily with the paralyzing failure of orthodox belief in the Low Calorie diet. It's the most logical one in theory. In practice, it's the most disconcerting and the least effective. It sets quotas, doses and portions but forgets that the people having to follow it are made of flesh and blood, emotions and instincts. The most motivated ones may manage to lose weight but all or almost all of them put it back on. If we don't act and act quickly, weight problems will become a devastating scourge.'

Deeply appalled that this strategy's patent failure was being denied, despite increasing statistical evidence every year, Dukan made a simple but extremely important discovery, which would remain the cornerstone of his approach and conviction: *the human diet's three basic food groups (proteins, carbohydrates and fats) are not equally responsible for weight gain.* Although fats and sugars are quick, high-energy fuels, proteins are not supposed to provide energy and it is difficult to make use of their calories.

Dukan then put forward the first diet based on protein-rich foods, obtaining un-hoped for results, which allowed him to add to it his liberating 'as much as you want' concept. Over the decades, building on this foundation, he has created a complete method whose main elements include:

- 100 foods (72 protein foods, 28 vegetables) of which you can eat as much as you want.
- A structured 4-step programme, starting with the strictest, shortest but tremendously effective phase and ending with freedom to eat what you want.
- Absolute priority is given to stabilizing the weight achieved.
- Exercise is vitally important with walking top of the list.
- Pleasure also plays a huge role, and therefore 1,200 recipes are available.
- By using 11 adjustment parameters a weight is identified that can be both achieved and maintained – the True Weight.

- Learn how to lose weight through the gradual introduction of food groups within the programme.

Nowadays, many health professionals and epidemiologists believe the Dukan Method to be the method best equipped to put a halt to the weight problems that are still on the increase the world over.

INDEX

Index

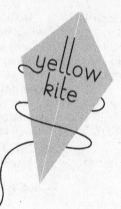

books to help you live a good life

Join the conversation and tell
us how you live a #goodlife

🐦 @yellowkitebooks
🅕 YellowKiteBooks
🅟 Yellow Kite Books
📷 YellowKiteBooks